Essentials
of the Earth
8th Edition

Expanded from the original Essentials of the Earth
(Essential Oils History, Overview and Reference Guide, 1st edition)
Updated August 2018

Published by:
Essentials of the Earth, LLC
info@EoEbooks.com

This book is intended as an informational guide. The essential oils and suggested application techniques described herein are meant to supplement, and not to be a substitute for, professional medical care or treatment. They should not be used to treat a serious ailment without prior consultation with a qualified healthcare professional.

ISBN 978-1-934711-00-2

8th edition, 1st printing, 2018
Printed in the United States of America

Special Cautions

The essential oils spoken of in this work are the natural oils extracted from different trees and plants from various locations on the earth. Many have been used by mankind for millenia for their helpful purposes in maintaining health. On the other hand, the information researched and reported in this book is NOT the result of modern scientific studies. This is a compilation of experiences and results noted by early authors, contemporary books and individuals (see page 31). It has NOT been scientifically verified or reviewed by medical professionals to establish the authenticity of the results. We urge anyone with a serious medical condition to utilize the expertise of professional medical experts.

Further, the process of growing and extracting essential oils is not a regulated industry. A great deal of variation can exist in an essential oil known by a common name but provided by different companies. We urge anyone using essential oils to seek for the highest quality and to be assured of this quality by the provider. This would include the provider identifying the location, growing conditions and harvesting techniques used. Also they should note the processing procedures that are used as well as modern testing techniques to verify the quality of their oils.

> **Please note:** Much of the information provided in this book is based on a compilation of the experiences of others who have used essential oils and has NOT been scientifically verified with clinical tests nor reviewed by medical experts. It is anecdotal information and should be treated as such. **If you have serious medical concerns or a life-threatening condition please seek immediate professional medical attention.** Essentials of the Earth, LLC does not claim that the information in this book will heal, cure or eliminate medical conditions and cannot be held liable for the use of essential oils to treat such.

Dedication

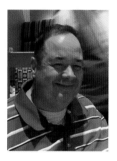

Robert Lyle James 1963 - 2018

Robert Lyle James had a passion and understanding of essential oils and was the inspiration and co-author of the very first edition of this Essentials of the Earth book. His desire to share with others led him to have and help with other ways to pass on valuable knowledge. Sharing websites were a favorite tool including a Google Group that he hosted for years. This became a key source of information for another sharing website EverythingEssential.me that helped many to find the value of essential oils in their lives.

His generous, caring and giving nature coupled with his sense of humor blessed us all. We will miss him and know that he is in the arms of his Savior and is sharing now with those in our Heavenly Home above.

CONTENTS

An Overview of Essential Oils

What are they?

Essential oils are the natural extracts of the life protecting fluids of natural vegetation. Plants develop their own protection against the pathogens in their environment which is stored as an oil. The oils are most commonly extracted from the plant material through steam distillation. Depending on the plant, this can be from the flowers, leaves, rind, resin, bark or roots of the plant. The oils are extracted in a highly concentrated form and can be used in a number of ways to protect and aide health.

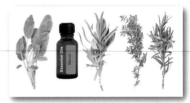

Many of these natural oils have some of the strongest antibacterial, antiviral and antifungal properties found today. In addition, many have aromatic properties that work with the human limbic system to stimulate powerful calming and balancing responses. Herbs, like ginger, have long been used to soothe the digestive system. Oils of these natural plants provide benefits in a concentrated, measurable and easily accessible form. Aromatherapy is a common term used for the application of essential oils for health benefits.

Are they proven?

Essential oils are some of the oldest and most powerful therapeutic agents know to man. As early as ancient Egypt, up to the time of Christ, through the dark ages and down to the twentieth century they have been used for their medicinal properties. In the early 1900's modern research got its start as French researchers began to explore and document their properties. This was soon followed by researchers and practitioners in Germany and England. Names like Valnet, Tisserand and Schnaubelt did foundational work and many of their findings provide the basis for the information and guidelines included in this compilation. Beyond

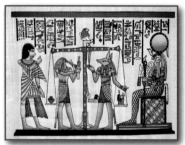

this, there are many contemporary experts who have contributed significant documented experiences upon which we have drawn. The work continues with many universities, research laboratories and individuals doing studies of these marvelous health-supporting products. Going to PubMed.com on the Internet and searching on the various essential oils and health concerns will reveal the interest, studies and findings that are happening every day.

Nature's Medicine Cabinet

With the world recognizing the benefits of "Going Green" it seems as though producers of many products from energy sources to cleaning compounds, from health antidotes to beauty treatments are recognizing what nature has had to offer for centuries. Alternative health conscious studies and products are turning to Mother Nature for more "green" products.

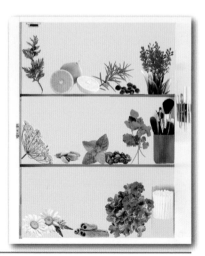

Essential oils lead the way! Man has known about nature's amazing antidotes for centuries. Now modern technology has made extraction, production and delivery of these possible. Powerful plant constituents are being used to make more potent products that can be effective in health, beauty and longevity.

The trend of going green in energy, beauty products and health alternatives has begun. It's time to jump on board the wagon and be a part of the new sustainable efforts in health, beauty and life.

What should I look for?

Like quality wine, different locations and different growing conditions provide the highest quality essential oils. The best frankincense comes from Oman, the best lemon from Italy and so forth. The methods of growing, harvesting and extracting the oils is critical. There are many sources of essential oils with a wide variety of prices. Finding a company that guarantees the quality of their oils is very important. They should provide assurance that they source their oils from the best locations in the world with documentation to confirm this and that growing and harvesting conditions are optimal. Beyond this there should be a guarantee that <u>every</u> batch of the essential oils is tested with the latest methods to assure quality, purity and potency.

As mentioned elsewhere the suggestions made in this book are based on experiences of those using the very high quality essential oils. Those using inferior quality oils should not expect the same positive results as recorded herein. The quality described above is the assurance you need to make your experiences using essential oils rewarding and repeatable.

How to Use Essential Oils

The use of essential oils is primarily a self-help model. Many conditions such as a cut, a bruise or a headache may find help with simple common sense use of the oils. An antibiotic oil directly on a cut, a drop of Peppermint on the forehead for a headache, etc. Other conditions may not be as straightforward and the experiences of others can give great insight.

This book shares the experiences of many to help the reader develop their own insight and positive experiences. With time and experience most come to understand their body and develop a sense for those oils and application techniques that will have positive impact.

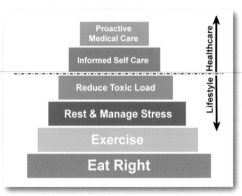

It is true that each person is unique and may respond to an oil in slightly different ways than others. This is why there will often be a number of oils and blends mentioned for a particular need in this publication. Different individuals will have more positive results with some oils and application methods than others or from one time to the next so it may be necessary to experiment to find your most effective combination.

The selection of an essential oil, blend or product is important but the application technique is also important. The oils may be applied or utilized in a variety of ways. These may be divided into three primary categories as described in the following paragraphs.

Inhalation

As the vapors of essential oils are inhaled they immediately travel to the limbic system of the brain where they have a profound affect on moods, emotions, alertness and other functions controlled by this central part of the brain. Inhalation also allows the antibacterial, antifungal and antiviral properties of the oils to be delivered directly to the respiratory organs. Inhalation techniques include:

Diffusion using ultrasonic and nebulizing atomization of essential oils in living and working spaces. Properly diffused oils are known to kill bacteria and virus, improve mental clarity, enhance or calm emotions and increase feelings of well-being. A well designed diffuser can fill a room, office or lobby with therapeutic aromatics in only minutes. Over longer periods of time these diffused oils strengthen the immune system, reduce mold and reduce unpleasant orders.

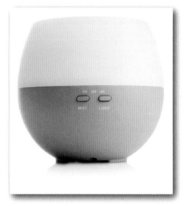

Direct Inhalation can be conveniently accomplished with a number of techniques including direct inhalation either from an essential oil bottle, the hands (using cup & inhale) or from a tissue cup. Another technique is to use self-made inhalers or spritz bottles with a suggested oil or blend. Steam tents or a T-shirt tent can help with respiratory issues and a cotton ball in an auto vent works well while traveling. (See more information on any of these techniques in the A to Z section.)

Topical

Topical application allows oils to quickly enter the bloodstream and circulate throughout the body. Logic often dictates where to apply an oil. Often applying directly to the affected area is most effective. The pressure points identified in acupressure or reflexology on the soles of the feet or palms of the hands have also proven effective places to apply oils. Direct topical application of the oils can be enhanced with other techniques as discussed below:

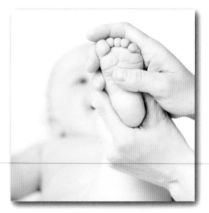

Massage techniques used on a local area or essential oils coupled with the work of a professional massage therapist (or massage practitioner) can enhance the benefits significantly. The Massage Blend Technique described in the A to Z section of this book is a great tool.

Massage for infants and young children can be very helpful. The bottoms of the feet are a highly effective pathway to their bodies. Care must be taken with their sensitive skin and protection from transfer of oils to the eyes should be used. Consider the chart in the chart section at the end of this book and study carefully more comprehensive sources before using this technique on babies and young children.

Compresses applied after topical application of oils using a warm or cold towel is often suggested to drive the oils deeper. For some situations warm is preferred while others will specify cold.

Baths and soakings can range from a local hand or foot bath to a full body bath with oils. Showers, sitz baths, jacuzzi and saunas can all couple with the benefits of essential oils.

Internal

Many high quality oils may be used internally to provide immediate help for oral, gastrointestinal and other concerns. Common techniques

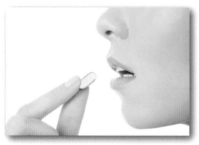

for internal use include adding the oils to capsules and taking orally, preparing and sipping teas, simply adding to water or juice or a drop under the tongue. There are some occasions that a suppository using a capsule or a syringe is suggested. Swishing oils in the mouth or using the oil pulling technique are types of internal/topical application that will be suggested by some. These are each described in more detail in the A to Z section of this book.

Most essential oils, if extracted and prepared properly, are safe for internal use. To verify this look for the FDA label of Supplemental Facts on the bottle. If this notation is present it indicates the oil is designated as GRAS (Generally Regarded as Safe) and may be used internally.

There are a few oils that are not recommended for internal use and will never have the FDA Supplemental Facts label. These are shown in the Safety Considerations section along with other important safety considerations when using oils.

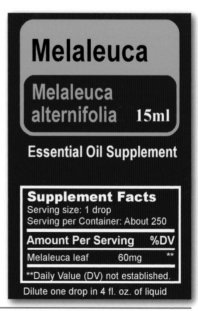

The Science and Synergy of Essential Oils

Science

There are many anecdotal stories of essential oils having very positive results for a variety of wellness situations and health concerns. Because they have been in use for liter-ally thousands of years, consider their continued use over time as research that is more substantial rather than anecdotal. Time has a way of being a natural filter; good things continue to be used while ineffective things fade into forgetfulness.

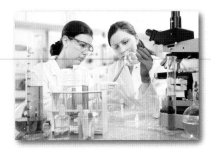

Beyond this, what does mod-ern science have to say? Kurt Schnaubelt, in his classical work *Medical Aromatherapy, Healing with Essential Oils,* gives an excellent synopsis of earlier researcher's studies and findings covering the period from the 1800's through the 1990's. He puts in perspective the scientific works of Gattefossé, Valnet, Tisserand, Belaiche and Franchomme as well as Pénoël whose laboratory testing identified the major properties of essential oils; antibacterial, antifungal, anti-parasitic, antiviral, etc. Oils were tested to show the actual levels of effectiveness of the various oils against differ-ent pathogens.

Research continues and is accelerating in our time. The Internet provides a valuable resource to research much of this activity. Simple searches can provide interesting results. From the 1990's there are these examples:

Bassett IB, et al. "A comparative study of tea-tree oil versus benzoyl peroxide in the treatment of acne." Med J Aust. 1990; 153(8): 455-8.

Buchbauer G, et al. "Aromatherapy: evidence for sedative effects of the essential oil of Lavender after inhalation." Z Naturforsch [C]. 1991; 46(11-12): 1067-72.

The above samples are just 2 of many from the 1990s and the pace of research has even quickened since. The author of *Nature's Living Energy: A Personal Guide to Using Essential Oils (2007)* asserts, "There are currently over 4,000 papers published on the effects of essential oils housed in the National Library of Medicine. Perusing only a few will help you understand a key principle. It is the complexity of essential oils that governs such profound effects physiologically and it is also their mystery yet to be fully discovered." That interest and discovery will lead to many more refined uses and more dramatic results.

Synergy

This is the interaction of two or more agents or forces that when combined produces a total effect that is greater than the sum of their individual parts. This is an important concept when using essential oils.

Synergy in blending: A unified marriage of the correct oils in proper proportions with harmonious frequencies is considered highly compatible and efficacious as a whole, as opposed to the benefit from an independent oil when used alone. Effective blends of certified pure therapeutic grade oils offer an exhilarating union that creates a highly effective outcome.

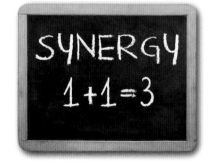

Application synergy: Coupling the essential oils with the best application technique can prove very valuable. Elsewhere are described various techniques such as diffusion, massage, baths, direct topical, ingestion, etc. Understand and select the best for each health concern.

Theistic Synergy: There are those that believe plants were placed on earth as our pharmacy and that accepting this divine background increases their faith in the benefits of essential oils. Often prayer and/ or meditation is used as a complementary, supportive measure. For many, the synergizing affects of prayer used simultaneously with other remedies offers some of the most effective helping opportunities.

Healthful Synergy: Synergy does not just apply to blending oils. There are other things that, when combined with oils, make them stronger and more effective. Defensive wellness programs, balanced nutrition, exercise and weight management all make essential oils more effective when necessary. The effectiveness of oils is also measurably enhanced as the body is cleansed. Detoxifying cleanses are described in the body of this book.

Safety Considerations

> **Please note:** Much of the information provided in this book is based on a compilation of the experiences of others who have used essential oils and has NOT been scientifically verified with clinical tests nor reviewed by medical experts. It is anecdotal information and should be treated as such. **For serious medical concerns please seek professional medical attention.**

Essential oils vary in their characteristics and each person is different in how they may respond to using them. Negative reactions are unusual but it is important to have an understanding of the characteristics of the various oils and any necessary precautions.

The most common unwanted result is skin irritation. To avoid this situation it is always prudent with topical applications to dilute oils with a carrier and if in doubt perform a basic skin test.

Basic Skin Test

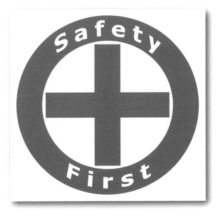

Place a very small amount of the essential oil on the inside of the elbow, underside of the forearm or wrist. After approximately 1 hour, check the area(s) for any type of reactition.

If an essential oil causes irritation, mixing the oil with a carrier or applying a carrier followed by the essential oil will usually make the oil usable. Undiluted oils are not likely to irritate the tough skin of the sole of the foot and will rapidly enter the body. Except in the case of a few "hot" oils such as Oregano, Clove, Thyme and Cinnamon Bark most users will not react to exceptionally high quality, pure oils and therefore they can be safely applied for a direct and powerful effect. This is one of many reasons to always use quality essential oils.

Basic Precautions for Using Essential Oils

Some Essential Oils Increase Photosensitivity. Photosensitivity is an increased sensitivity of the skin to radiant energy or light such as natural sunlight, sunlamps or other sources of UV rays causing the skin to sunburn more easily than usual. Topical application of certain oils to exposed skin further intensifies this effect. An adverse response may appear within minutes, hours or days after first application and exposure. These oils are primarily citrus oils and include Angelica, Bergamot, Grapefruit, Lemon, Lime, Orange, Tangerine and Wild Orange. In addition to sunburn, this may result in a dark pigmentation or a rash on the skin. Bergamot contains bergaptene, a dominant photosensitizer and can cause severe reactions. When using photosensitizing oil, wait at least 6 - 12 hours before exposing skin to UV rays and be especially careful with Bergamot.

Use Care with Infants and Individuals with Sensitive Skin. Quite frankly, some people just have sensitive skin. Common sense should be used. Increased watchfulness should be used when treating infants, young children and the elderly. Their skin is much more sensitive and susceptible to irritation, burning or stinging sensations. Using an effective carrier oil will protect sensitive skin against irritation.

Use Care with Eyes, Ears, etc. Never apply oils directly to the eyes or ear canal. After application, be attentive to things like rubbing the eyes, areas around the eye, eyelids, handling contact lenses or touching the interior of one's nose. The skin is also quite sensitive and prone to irritation around the genitals and mucous membranes.

Use Care When Applying Oils to Infants and Children. After application young children should be supervised to prevent transfer of oils from application areas to his or her eyes (cross contamination). The best precaution is to clothe application areas until the oils have been sufficiently absorbed.

Pregnancy. Aromatherapists generally agree that oils topically (externally) applied in ordinary amounts are not harmful to a developing fetus. However, pregnant women may want to consult a physician or aromatherapy practitioner prior to using essential oils. If there are specific oils that pregnant women should be concerned about it will be noted on the oil bottle from most reputable suppliers. *See the safety charts on pages following for specific recommendations.*

Breast Feeding. Some report decreased milk supply with Peppermint, others do not. To err on the side of caution Peppermint and blends using Peppermint (Digestive Blend, Encouraging Blend, Metabolic Blend, Soothing Blend) should be limited if milk production is at risk. Also some point out that what mothers ingest is passed through to breast milk so "hot" oils or certain tastes may affect some infants and toxins eliminated during a mothers detoxification can be passed to breast milk.

Critical Health Conditions. Persons with epilepsy, high blood pressure or other critical health conditions can benefit from essential oils. By the same token, there are a few oils that are contra-indicated for these conditions. When in doubt it is recommended that one consult a healthcare or aromatherapy professional when addressing these serious conditions. *See the safety charts on pages following for specific recommendations.*

Oils Not Suitable for Use in Aromatherapy. Caution or consultation with a qualified professional should be used before using wormwood, pennyroyal, camphor, sassafras, onion, bitter almond and horseradish. Ruta gravenolens or rue essential oil is classified as poisonous to humans and should not be used.

A Little Goes a Long Way. There is a reason for the reducer insert in top of oil bottles. True, high quality essential oils are pure concentrates. The higher quality the oil the more potent it is and smaller amounts are required. A little goes a long way.

Internal Use. Many exceptionally high quality essential oils are safe for ingesting; some are not. Additionally, inexpensive, low quality oils are not. The chart following will note if a very high quality brand of each oil is typically GRAS, that is, "generally regarded as safe" as a food additive by the FDA. *In addition each bottle of oil that is safe for internal consumption will include a supplemental facts label.* Most suggestions for using oils internally, especially for children, will include techniques for diluting them with water, agave, honey, juice or a carrier oil. Also most suggest never using internally with infants.

Keep Out of Reach of Children. Treat essential oils as what they are - a natural medicine. Oils can be painful used in the eyes, caustic to sensitive skin without a carrier or harmful if large quantities of the wrong oil are ingested.

Essential Oil and Bath Water. One common application method is use of full body, foot or hand baths. When using undiluted oil in bath water, disperse the oil by agitating the water. You can also use a dispersing agent such as unscented, chemically free bath gel or hand lotion or Epsom salt.

Oils and Low Grade Plastics. Single oils and blends are delivered in quality glass containers for a reason. Many oils will soften or dissolve plastics if left in contact with them for some length of time. Using oils diluted in a spritz bottle or inhaler made of plastic will have no ill effects but it would not be wise to transfer an oil from its own bottle to a plastic container for storage or even to put a few drops of lemon in a low grade plastic water bottle for drinking during the day.

Many Oils Are Flammable. Keep them clear of open flame, sparks or other fire hazards.

Safety Charts

The charts following are summaries of information gleaned from respected authors regarding the safety characteristics of most common oils and blends. The GRAS and other information is based on a very high quality essential oil brand and may not apply to all sources of essential oils. The legend below explains the terms for both charts.

Legend for Blends and Oils Charts		
Skin sensitivity	Mild	Most find these oils mild to use without dilution.
	Skin test	Can be a skin irritant. Use a skin test and dilute if necessary.
	Dilute	Can be a strong skin irritant. Dilute with a carrier oil.
Photo-sensitive	Yes, use care	May react to sunlight or UV rays. Avoid sunlight or UV exposure 6 - 12 hours after topical use on exposed skin.
GRAS	Yes	Can be used internally if oil supplier has the "supplements" label on the bottle that indicates it is certified by the FDA as "Generally Regarded As Safe."
	Not internal	Not recommended for use internally.
Pregnancy	Use	Most find these acceptable to use.
	Use/care (use with care)	Consider dilution with carrier oil. Avoid repeated application over long periods of time.
	Consult	Consult a qualified aromatherapist or physician before using.

(Also see notes following charts.)

Essential Oils Blends Safety Chart

Oil Blends	Skin sensitivity	Photo-sensitive	GRAS (internal use)	Preg-nancy
Anti-Aging Blend	Mild	No	Not internal	Use care
Blend for Women	Mild	No	Not internal	Use
Calming Blend	see Restful Blend			
Cellular Complex	Skin test	No	Yes	Consult
Centering Blend	Mild	Yes, use care	Not internal	Consult
Cleansing Blend	Mild	No	Not internal	Use
Comforting Blend	Skin test	No	n/a	Consult
Courage Blend for Children	Skin test	Yes, use care	Not internal	for children
Detoxification Blend	Mild	Yes, use care	Yes	Consult
Digestive Blend	Mild	No	Yes	Consult
Encouraging Blend	Skin test	Yes, use care	n/a	Consult
Enlightening Blend	Mild	Yes, use care	Not internal	Consult
Focus Blend	Mild	No	Not internal	Use care
Focus Blend for Children	Skin test	No	Not internal	for children
Fortifying Blend	Skin test	No	Not internal	Consult
Grounding Blend	Mild	No	Not internal	Use
Grounding Blend for Children	Skin test	No	Not internal	for children
Inspiring Blend	Skin test	No	n/a	Consult
Invigorating Blend	Mild	Yes, use care	Not internal	Use

Joyful Blend	Mild	Yes, use care	Not internal	Use
Massage Blend	Mild	No	Not internal	Use
Metabolic Blend	Mild	No	Yes	Consult
Monthly B for Women	Mild	No	Not internal	Consult
Outdoor Blend	Mild	No	Not internal	Use care
Peaceful Child Blend	Mild	No	Not internal	n/a
Protective Blend	Mild	No	Yes	Consult
Protective Blend for Children	Skin test	No	Not internal	for children
Protective Blend+	capsule	No	Yes	Consult
Reassuring Blend	Skin test	No	n/a	Consult
Renewing Blend	Skin test	No	n/a	Consult
Respiratory Blend	Mild	No	Not internal	Use
Restful Blend	Mild	No	Not internal	Consult
Restful Blend for Children	Skin test	No	Not internal	for children
Seasonal Blend	capsule	No	Yes	Use care
Soothing Blend	Mild	No	Not internal	Consult
Soothing Blend for Children	Skin test	No	Not internal	for children
Steadying Blend	Mild	No	Not internal	Consult
Tension Blend	Mild	No	Not internal	Use care
Topical Blend	Mild	No	Not internal	Use care
Uplifting Blend	Skin test	Yes, use care	n/a	Consult
Yarrow-Pomegranate	Skin test	No	Yes	Consult

Single Oil Safety Chart

Single Oils	Skin sensitivity	Photo-sensitive	GRAS (internal use)	Pregnancy
Arborvitae	Mild	No	Not internal	Use care
Basil	Mild	No	Yes	Consult
Bergamot*	Skin test	Yes, Use care*	Yes	Use
Birch*	Dilute	No	Not internal	Avoid
Black Pepper	Skin test	No	Yes	Use
Blue Tansy	Mild	No	Not interna	Consult
Cardamom	Mild	No	Yes	Use
Cassia	Dilute	No	Yes	Consult
Cedarwood	Skin test	No	Not internal	Use care
Cilantro	Mild	No	Yes	Consult
Cinnamon Bark	Dilute	No	Yes	Consult
Clary Sage	Mild	No	Yes	Consult
Clove	Dilute	No	Yes	Use care
Copaiba	Skin test	No	Yes	Consult
Coriander	Mild	No	Yes	Use
Cumin	Mild	Yes, Use care	Yes	Use care
Cypress	Mild	No	Not internal	Use care
Dill	Mild	No	check oil source	Avoid
Douglas Fir	Mild	No	Not internal	Consult
Elemi	Skin test	No	check oil source	Consult
Eucalyptus	Skin test	No	Not internal	Use care
Fennel	Skin test	No	Yes	Consult
Frankincense	Mild	No	Yes	Use
Geranium	Skin test	No	Yes	Use

Single Oils	Skin sensitivity	Photo-sensitive	GRAS (internal use)	Pregnancy
Ginger	Skin test	No	Yes	Use care
Grapefruit	Mild	Yes, Use care	Yes	Use
Green Mandarin	Mild	Yes, mild	Yes	Use
Helichrysum	Mild	No	Yes	Use
Jasmine	Mild	No	Yes	Consult
Juniper Berry	Mild	No	Yes	Consult
Lavender	Mild	No	Yes	Use
Lemon	Mild	Yes, Use care	Yes	Use
Lemongrass	Skin test	No	Yes	Use care
Lime	Skin test	Yes, Use care	Yes	Use
Litsea	Skin test	No	check oil source	Consult
Magnolia	Skin test	No	check oil source	Use
Manuka	Skin test	No	check oil source	Consult
Marjoram	Mild	No	Yes	Consult
Melaleuca	Mild	No	Yes	Use care
Melissa	Mild	No	Yes	Use
Myrrh	Mild	No	Yes	Use care
Neroli	Mild	No	Not internal	Use
Oregano*	Dilute	No	Yes	Consult
Patchouli	Mild	No	Yes	Use
Peppermint*	Skin test	No	Yes	Use care
Petitgrain	Skin test	No	Yes	Consult
Pink Pepper	Mild	No	Yes	Use

Single Oils	Skin sensitivity	Photo- sensitive	GRAS (internal use)	Pregnancy
Ravensara	Mild	No	check oil source	Consult
Roman Chamomile	Mild	No	Yes	Use
Rose	Mild	No	Yes	Use care
Rosemary	Mild	No	Yes	Consult
Sandalwood	Mild	No	Yes	Use
Siberian Fir	Mild	No	Yes	Consult
Spearmint	Skin test	No	Yes	Consult
Spikenard	Mild	No	Not internal	Consult
Star Anise*	Skin test	No	Yes	Avoid
Tangerine	Mild	Yes, Use care	Yes	Use
Thyme	Dilute	No	Yes	Consult
Turmeric*	Mild	No	Yes	Consult
Vetiver	Mild	No	Yes	Consult
White Fir	Mild	No	Not internal	Use care
Wild Orange	Mild	Yes, Use care	Yes	Use
Wintergreen* (Gaul-theria fragrantissima)	Skin test*	No	Not internal	Avoid
Wintergreen* (Gaul-theria procumbens)	Skin test*	No	Not internal	Avoid
Yarrow	Dilute	No	check oil source	Avoid
Ylang Ylang	Mild	No	Yes	Use
*see further notes following				

Special Notes Related to the Safety Charts

* Bergamot

    More photosensitive than other citrus oils.

* Birch and Wintergreen:

    Can be irritants or even toxic at high levels.
    Do not use on children or during pregnancy.

* Oregano

    If taking internally use a maximum 2 weeks; then rest the body (stop) 1-2 weeks before continuing.

* Peppermint

    Topically has a strong cooling sensation. Use extreme caution with infants.

* Star Anise

    Essential Oil Safety (Tisserand/Young) notes these Contraindications: pregnancy, breastfeeding, endometriosis, estrogen-dependent cancers, children under 5. Also these Cautions (oral): diabetes medication, anticoaulant medication, major surgery, peptic ulcer, hemophilia and other bleeding disorders.

* Turmeric

    Possible interaction with diabetic medications.

Sensitivity:

    Please be aware that some people are very sensitive and may experience a reaction to the mildest of oils. Use a skin test if there is any question. (*see* Basic Skin Test earlier in this section of the book.)

Epilepsy:

    Avoid Basil, Birch, Dill, Fennel, Rosemary and Wintergreen.

    Also mentioned from other sources and experiences are these oils to avoid or to use with care: Arborvitae, Camphor, Eucalyptus, Fennel, Galbanum, Hyssop, Nutmeg, Pennyroyal, Sage, Savin, Spike Lavender (not the common Lavender angustifolia), Tansy (not to be confused with Blue Tansy), Tarragon, Thuja, Thujone, Turpentine and Wormwood.

    Note: Soothing Blend has Camphor and Wintergreen and Protective Blend has Eucalyptus and Rosemary.

High blood pressure:

Avoid Rosemary and Thyme.

Grapefruit oil has not been known to interfere with blood pressure medications. It has been pointed out that the compound naringin, found in the fruit of grapefruit, causes problems with prescription medications by interfering with or amplifying the body's ability to absorb the drugs. Naringin is not present in the rind of the grapefruit and hence not in Grapefruit essential oil.

Please note: Much of the information provided in this book is based on a compilation of the experiences of others who have used essential oils and has NOT been scientifically verified with clinical tests nor reviewed by medical experts. It is anecdotal information and should be treated as such. **If you have serious medical concerns or a life-threatening condition please seek immediate professional medical attention.** Essentials of the Earth, LLC does not claim that the information in this book will heal, cure or eliminate medical conditions and cannot be held liable for the use of essential oils to treat such.

Information Sources

This book is an expanded edition of *The Essential Oil History, Overview and Reference Guide*, first published in 2008. After three printings of this first edition we chose to expand our database with additional contemporary sources and broaden the information in the book. We continue to update it regularly.

Following is a brief description of the database and other sources used for this edition of the book:

1) A database listing 1300 health concern terms with over 540 unique health concerns and the essential oils recommended by both early essential oils authors and contemporary sources. Data compiled in the database comes from:

Jean Valnet, MD, *The Practice of Aromatherapy, A Classic Compendium of Plant Medicines & Their Healing Properties*

Kurt Schnaubelt, *Medical Aromatherapy, Healing with Essential Oils*

Sampling of Health Concern Database

Major and Sub Health Concerns	see...	Mentioned (Factor = 1 or 2)	Suggested (Factor = 3 or 4)	Preferred (Factor greater than
abscess		Lavender(C), Melaleuca(C),		
skin abscess	skin conditions		(C),	
tooth abcess	teeth conditions			
abuse	emotional conditions			
achalasia	swallowing conditions			
acid reflux (heart burn)		Eucalyptus(C), Lemon(C), Wild Orange(C),	Basil(EC), Black pepper(E), Coriander(C), Roman chamomile(C), Sandalwood(C),	Ginger(C), Peppermint(C), (C),
GERD				
acne		Bergamot(E), Cypress(C), Frankincense(C), Lemon(C), Lemongrass(C), Melaleuca(EC), Patchouli(C), Peppermint(E), Thyme(C), Vetiver(C),	Geranium(C), Rosemary(EC), (C),	Lavender(EC), Sandalwoo
pimples				
ADD/ADHD (attention deficit disorder)		Basil(C), Lavender(C),	Frankincense(C), Patchouli(C), (C), (C), (C),	Vetiver(C), (C),
addictions				

Robert B. Tisserand, *The Art of Aromatherapy, The Healing and Beautifying Properties of the Essential Oils of Flowers and Herbs*

Nature's Living Energy and notes from the author's seminars

Please recognize that each writer had available to them different collections of essential oils and possibly not the quality that is presently available. These are reasons why one expert's suggestions do not always agree with another.

2) Experiences and testimonials shared with us by those utilizing our information and with a desire to share their own personal experiences.

3) Experiences and suggestions from contemporary experts both published in print and on the internet.

4) Modern research results from PubMed and other scientific sources.

How to Use the A to Z Guide

Categories

This book is arranged as a mini-encyclopedia of fingertip information for choosing and applying essential oils. The 800+ entries are arranged alphabetically and include five specific categories with different highlighting/images.

Health concerns - These entries have a blue headline and include the essential oils, blends and essential oils inspired products with application techniques that have been found helpful in the experiences of others for the specific condition.

> ### *Acne* (and pimples)
>
> **Oils:** Geranium^C, Melaleuca^EC **Blends:** Cleansing Blend^C, Topical Blend^C
>
> 2 times daily, after cleansing skin, 3-5 drops of

The other four catagories all have a dark orange headline. These include Essential Oils, Blends, Products and Glossary Terms:

Essential Oils - Each of the entries for essential oils includes the common name, the Latin name, a picture of the plant, some of the most noteworthy properties and common health concerns helped with this oil based on the experiences of others.

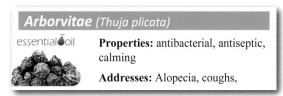

> ### *Arborvitae* (Thuja plicata)
>
> essential oil
>
> **Properties:** antibacterial, antiseptic, calming
>
> **Addresses:** Alopecia, coughs,

Blends - Blends are a combination of essential oils mixed together for the synergistic effect this combination can deliver. The brief description includes the essential oils in the blend and the health concerns helped based on the experiences of others.

> ### *Calming Blend* (can help give a serene attitude)
>
> essential●oils
> **Blend**
>
> **Ingredients:** Lavender, Roman Chamomile, Sandalwood
>
> **Addresses:** Anxiety, calming, induces

Products - There are a number of essential oil-based products that are often mentioned by experts and others for their benefits. Included in this book are many of the most frequently mentioned products and a brief description of their ingredients and common uses.

> ### *Cellular Complex Blend Capsules*
>
> essential●oils
> **Product**
>
> The same as the Cellular Complex Blend with 8 drops of the blend in a single vegetarian softgel.

Glossary terms - Some terms or abbreviations used throughout the book may not be familiar to those new to essential oils. Many such common terms and abbreviations are interspersed in the A to Z section with a brief explanation to help those new to using oils.

> ### *Carrier oil*   *see also* Lotions
>
>
> De**inition**
>
> A mild, light oil that may be used to mix with an essential oil for those with sensitive skin and/or to assist in massaging oils into the skin.

Color Codes and Superscripts

In the blue Health Concern entries the essential oils suggested are color coded and some include superscripts. The suggested oils are color coded to reflect how often they were suggested by the experts and the superscripts, in an abbreviated way, indicate who made the suggestion.

Color codes:

Green	Preferred or frequently suggested.
Gold	Suggested as an alternative or a supplemental oil.
Red	Also mentioned or noted as successful for some.

Superscript codes:

Superscript E (Lemon^E)	Indicates this oil was mentioned by at least one of the early experts Valnet, Schnaubelt or Tisserand.
Superscript C (Lavender^C)	Indicates this oil or blend was mentioned by at least one of the contemporary experts.
No superscript	This oil or blend suggestion is based on the repeated experiences of others. (Some health concerns, for example ADD, were not recognized in the earlier times hence not reviewed by the early experts.)

Terms and cross references

The primary names we have used for the health concerns in this book are the names commonly used in everyday conversations. There are many synonyms, acronyms and variants (closely related terms) for many health concerns. Examples of how these are entered in the A to Z section are included below followed with a short summary:

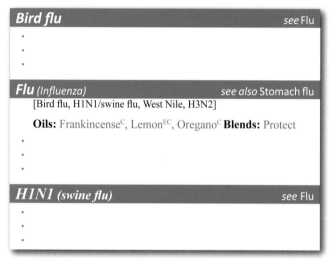

Bird flu   *see* Flu

- .
- .
- .

Flu *(Influenza)*   *see also* Stomach flu

[Bird flu, H1N1/swine flu, West Nile, H3N2]

Oils: Frankincense[C], Lemon[EC], Oregano[C] **Blends:** Protect

- .
- .
- .

H1N1 *(swine flu)*   *see* Flu

- .
- .
- .

Summary

- Paranthesis ( ) generally indicate a synonym.

- Square bracket [ ] generally indicates a variant or a related term. The terms in square brackets indicates there are, in this case, variants of the general term Flu that may be helped with information given in this general catagory of Flu.

- *"see"* points to the primary name where information is available.

- *"see also"* indicates there may be information of further interest to the reader in the referenced location.

Special notes on Oils and Blend Names

Why so many oils? Some have asked, "Why are there so many oils suggested for some conditions?" This is because different oils have overlapping properties and each person's body can respond to an oil in a slightly different way. Hence we have tried to include a broad range of the suggestions we have compiled. We recognize that with the "self help" model many essential oils users will experiment with these different alternatives to find an optimum outcome suited to them.

Generic blend names. Essential oil blends have names given to them by their supplier. In this publication, the names for blends and products are generic or descriptive and not the brand name of any one company. Tables of generic names vs. brand names can ususally be found online at sites associated with the various essential oils suppliers or we can help. Email us at info@eoebooks.com.

Notes:

_____

_____

_____

_____

_____

_____

_____

_____

_____

_____

_____

_____

_____

_____

_____

_____

_____

Legend: Preferred, Suggested, Consider

The A to Z Guide

Abscess *(skin, throat, tooth)*

Oils: Melaleuca[C], Oregano **Blends:** Protective Blend[C]

Skin: 2-3 drops Melaleuca, Protective Blend or diluted Oregano to area every 1/2-1 hour. Dilute if necessary or add Lemon to lessen burning.

Throat: 3 drops each Lemon or Protective Blend in mouthful of water, gargle 15-20 sec, swallow. Younger children 2 drops each Lemon and Protective Blend to spoonful of applesauce, swallow slowly.

Tooth: Oil pull Protective Blend or 2 drops each Clove (and Oregano for very bad conditions and very tough person), 2 Tbsp FCO, 2-3x daily. Brush with Protective Blend toothpaste 2x daily. Additional protection 2-4 drops each Protective Blend and Oregano in capsule daily.

Other oils: Clove, Frankincense, Helichrysum, Lavender[C], Lemon, Roman Chamomile **Blends:** Cleansing Blend

Absolute

 On a description of some oils or oils in a blend they will be noted as an "absolute" and not an "essential oil". The difference is that an essential oil almost always uses a process of extraction using steam (water based) or pressing. An absolute oil has used chemical solvents to extract the oil from the plant. This can then leave a trace of these solvents in the oil making it less desirable for health uses. The process is typically used for extracting oils for perfumes. Some flowers do not lend themselves to steam distillation and are best processed in this way. The chemical solvent process can be refined to minimize the trace chemicals remaining.

Acceptance
see Emotional strength

Achalasia
see Swallowing difficulty

Acid Reflux
see Heartburn

Acne *(and pimples)*

Oils: Geranium^C, Lavender^{EC}, Melaleuca^{EC}, Sandalwood^{EC} **Blends/ Products:** Cleansing Blend^C, EVCO, Topical Blend^C

2 times daily, after cleansing skin, 3-5 drops of Extra Virgin Coconut Oil in palm of the hand with 3-4 drops of the essential oil or blend. Pat onto affected area and leave on skin. The oils found most effective are shown above. (Some find Topical Blend strong and dilute or use Geranium and Melaleuca.)

From the experiences of others it is noted that different skin types will have more positive results with different oils so it may be necessary to experiment to find the best combination.

Note: Skin issues may indicate a need for internal cleansing. Adding 1-2 drops Lemon essential oil to your drinking water throughout the day is an excellent, gentle natural cleanse.

Other oils: Birch^C, Cedarwood^{EC}, Copaiba^C, Frankincense^C, Helichrysum^C, Juniper Berry^{EC}, Lemon^C, Lemongrass^C, Manuka^C, Petitgrain^C, Rosemary^{EC}, Yarrow^C **Blends:** Protective Blend

Acute inflammation
see Inflammation

ADD/ADHD *(attention deficit disorder)*

Oils: Clary Sage, Frankincense^C, Lavender^C, Vetiver^C, Ylang Ylang **Blends/Products:** Basic Vitality Supplements, Focus Blend, Grounding Blend^C, Peaceful Child Blend, Restful Blend

Focus Blend is a special blend prepared to enhance focus and support clear thought processes.

Frankincense stimulates the limbic system of the brain, Lavender is calming and relaxing to nervous system, Grounding Blend is detoxifying while promoting courage and self-esteem, Vetiver is calming and relaxing with inhalation and Clary Sage is uplifting and may help with depression. Basic Vitality Supplements for nutritional balance for proper brain function.

Legend: Preferred, Suggested, Consider

Apply to bottoms of the feet at bedtime and in the mornings. Remember a tender touch and quality time is important. Prepare an oils necklace to wear during the day. Apply to crown of head if there is a bad experience.

(Note: Many with these disorders are very sensitive to odors/touch, do not force application of oils if it is a negative experience. Some have success letting the child choose their own oils.)

Some have had success with a simple blend of Frankincense and Vetiver, others with the blend known as Peaceful Child applied to bottoms of feet and brain/spinal reflexology points of feet after morning shower.

Other oils: Basil[C], Dill[C], Marjoram, Patchouli[C] **Blends:** Invigorating Blend[C], Joyful Blend[C]

Addictions

[Alcohol, Drugs, Sugar, Tobacco]

Use an inhaler with oils of choice and breathe deeply when cravings appear. Topically apply to chest, wrists and/or bottom of feet. For eating addictions using Grapefruit or Metabolic Blend, add 3-7 drops to glass of water or in capsule 3-4x daily. For tobacco addiction transfer a drop of Cassia or Cinnamon Bark from finger to tongue.

General:

- Nutritional foundation: Basic Vitality Supplements
- Cravings: Cilantro, Cinnamon Bark, Clove[C], Grapefruit[C], Peppermint, Grounding Blend, Restful Blend[C]
- Anxiety: Lavender[C], Ylang Ylang[C], Grounding Blend , Restful Blend[C]
- Withdrawal: Lavender[C], Grapefruit[C], Marjoram[C], Sandalwood[C], Wild Orange[C], other citrus oils

Specific recommendations:

- Alcohol: Helichrysum[C], Rosemary[C], Cleansing Blend[C], Restful Blend[C]
- Caffeine: Basil, Metabolic Blend
- Drugs: Grapefruit, Roman Chamomile, Cleansing Blend[C], Restful Blend[C] **(Marijuana: Basil)**
- Energy drinks: Grapefruit, Energy & Stamina Complex
- Food: Grapefruit, Metabolic Blend

- **Pornography:** Frankincense, Helichrysum, Cleansing Blend
- **Sex:** Geranium, Sandalwood, Blend for Women, Monthly Blend for Women[C]
- **Sugar:** Grapefruit, Cleansing Blend[C], Metabolic Blend, Restful Blend[C]
- **Tobacco:** Black Pepper[C], Clove[C], Protective Blend[C]
- **Workaholic:** Basil[C], Geranium[C], Lavender[C], Marjoram[C], Wild Orange, Ylang Ylang

Addison's Disease *see* Adrenal Conditions and Autoimmune Diseases

Adenoids

Oils: Lemon **Blends:** Protective Blend, Respiratory Blend

Moderate swelling: 2-3 drops Protective Blend on bottoms of feet 2-3 times daily. Diffuse Respiratory Blend at bedtime.

Acute: Supplement Protective Blend with Oregano (or Cypress or Rosemary) for feet and apply topically diluted around and below ears. Dilute for small children. Diffuse Respiratory Blend and Eucalyptus (mix or rotate) at bedtime.

Other oils: Cypress, Eucalyptus, Grapefruit, Oregano, Peppermint, Rosemary **Blends:** Cleansing Blend

Adrenal conditions *(Adrenal fatigue or insufficiency)*

[Addison's disease, Cushing's syndrome, Schmidt's syndrome]

Oils: Basil[C], Clove[C], Geranium[EC], Rosemary[C] **Blends/Products:** Basic Vitality Supplements, Detoxification Blend/Detoxification Complex, Joyful Blend[C]

Immediate relief: 1-2 drops Clove and 1 drop Rosemary (or Coriander, Cypress, Geranium) topically over kidney area (lower back on each side of spine), follow with warm compress. Dilute with FCO for sensitive skin.

Long term: Basic Vitality Supplements, Detoxification Blend cleanse (see detoxification), Metabolic Blend to balance metabolism, lots of water with 1-2 drops Lemon per glass.

Other oils:

In General: Coriander, Cypress, Lavender, Ylang Ylang, Metabolic Blend, Restful Blend[C]

Adrenal failure: Geranium[E]

Adrenal insufficiency: Lemon[C], Melaleuca[C], Oregano[C], Joyful Blend[C]

Cushing's syndrome: Basil[C], Lemon[C]

Aerophagy bloating (bloating from swallowing air)   see Bloating

Age Spots (liver spots)

Oils: Frankincense, Lavender, Myrrh **Blends/Products:** Detoxification Blend/Detoxification Complex

Cleanse liver with Detoxification Blend/Detoxification Complex (*see* Detoxification) plus equal parts Frankincense, Lavender, Myrrh with EVCO applied topically daily.

Other oils: Manuka[C] **Blends/Products:** Basic Vitality Supplements, GI Cleansing Formula, Topical Blend, Probiotic Defense Formula

Agitation   see Irritability

AIDS (HIV or acquired immune deficiency syndrome)

Oils: Melissa[C] **Blends/Products:** Basic Vitality Supplements[C], Protective Blend[C]

The literature indicates no antiviral agents have yet been found that will defeat HIV but some suggest it may help to strengthen the immune system with a drop of Melissa and Protective Blend applied to the roof of the mouth daily. Couple this with healthy diet, exercise and Basic Vitality Supplements.

- Strengthen the immune system: Massage Blend
- Relieve stress and depression: Grounding Blend[C], Massage Blend, Lavender or Restful Blend with diffusing, cup & inhale or a Massage Blend Technique.

Other associated health concerns: Essential oils may help someone with a weakened immune system deal with pathogens.

- Candida infections (depending on the strength and tolerance of the individual):

Lemon^C (mild, easily tolerable)
Protective Blend^C (strong, tolerable)
Melaleuca (strong, reasonably tolerable)
Oregano^C (very strong, hot, usually requires diluting)

Esophagus, trachea, lungs: Consider diffusing, cup & inhale or capsules.
Oral: Consider oil pulling.
Vaginal or rectal: Oral capsules or rectal suppositories.
- Bacterial infections: Frankincense^C, Lavender, Melaleuca.
  Respiratory: Capsules or cup & inhale.
  Skin: Topical.
- Herpes simplex: Melaleuca should be applied neat or with a 50% carrier dilution. Apply topically to the outbreak area.

Other oils: Clove^C, Helichrysum^C

Air quality

Oils: Respiratory Blend, Eucalyptus^C, Lemon^C **Blends:** Cleansing Blend^C, Protective Blend

Diffuse blends/oils daily 2-3 hours. Rotate blends/oils periodically to address broader range of pathogens.
Disinfect: Eucalyptus, Protective Blend, Cleansing Blend, Lemon
Pleasant atomosphere: Invigorating Blend, Wild Orange, your favorite
Mood: Lavender, Joyful Blend, Restful Blend
Congestion: Respiratory Blend, Eucalyptus
Insomnia: Lavender, Restful Blend

10-15 drops Protective Blend or other oils to the filter in AC/Heater duct system when changing or more often if a diffuser is not available.

Other oils: Eucalyptus, Lavender, Melaleuca, Peppermint^C, Sandalwood

Air travel with oils

Oils: Frankincense, Lavender, Lemon, Melaleuca, Oregano, Peppermint
Blends/Products: Digestive Blend, Protective Blend, Protective Blend Throat Drops, Respiratory Blend, Soothing Blend

Basic oils above provide for most emergency situations while traveling.

Legend: Preferred, Suggested, Consider

The TSA Regulations Liquids Rule (2016) reads:

> You are allowed to bring a quart-sized bag of liquids, aerosols, gels, creams and pastes in your carry-on bag and through the checkpoint. These are limited to travel-sized containers that are 3.4 ounces (100 milliliters) or less per item. Placing these items in the small bag and separating from your carry-on baggage facilitates the screening process. Pack items that are in containers larger than 3.4 ounces or 100 milliliters in checked baggage.

The 15 ml essential oil bottles are 1/2 oz and a 1 quart zip lock holds a large number of bottles.

Alcohol   see Addictions

Alcohol (chemical)   see Chemical constituents

Aldehydes   see Chemical constituents

Alertness   see Mental acuity

Allergic reactions to essential oils   see Detoxification

Occasionally someone has a reaction to using essential oils. This can result in an uncomfortable rash or other reaction. Multiple scenarios can lead to this situation.

The person has very sensitive skin and reacts to topical application of the oils. This can be easily alleviated by diluting the essential oil with a carrier oil usually without lessening the effectiveness.

Using essential oils has triggered a Herxheimer reaction that may result in a rash or other external manifestation. For more information on this go to Herxheimer Reaction under Detoxification.

If the person is using inexpensive, low quality essential oils this can cause a reaction. Some inexpensive oils have additives that can cause adverse reactions. Use only high quality essential oils and blends.

Allergies
see also Food allergies and Food intolerance

[Dander, Dust, Hay fever, Mold, Pets, Pollen]

Oils: Lavender[C], Lemon[C], Peppermint[C] **Blends:** Seasonal Blend[C]

Airborne allergens: Take Seasonal Blend capsules every 3-4 hours to relieve symptoms or use oils individually every 3-4 hours in one of the following ways: 1) Put 2 drops Lavender and Lemon with 2-4 drops Peppermint in a capsule take internally. 2) For those bolder, mix the oils in a glass with a mouthful of juice or water, swish 10-20 sec in the mouth and swallow. 3) Mix a half portion in palms of hands; rub together, cup and inhale deeply for several seconds. It is best to start protocol as soon as allergies are felt or anticipated for quickest relief.

Other oils: Basil[C], Blue Tansy[EC], Lemongrass[C], Manuka[C], Melaleuca[C], Siberian Fir[C], Spikenard[C] **Blends:** Cleansing Blend[C], Protective Blend[C], Respiratory Blend[C], Turmeric[C]

Molds/fungus: Place several drops of Melaleuca, Lemongrass, Cleansing Blend or Protective Blend on an air intake filter in home. Diffuse any of the oils mentioned.

Dust mites, lice, fleas: Make 5% water spritz of Basil, Lemongrass or other oils, spray on bedding daily.

Alopecia
see Baldness

ALS *(Lou Gehrig's disease)*

Oils: Frankincense[C], Myrrh, Peppermint, Sandalwood[C], White Fir
Blends/Products: Basic Vitality Supplements, Cellular Complex Blend[C], Grounding Blend[C], Massage Blend, Restful Blend[C], Soothing Blend

Strengthen body: Basic Vitality Supplements, wholesome foods, eliminate alcohol, tobacco, carbonated drinks, high sugar content, etc.

Strengthen immune system: The Massage Blend Technique up to 2x daily.

Strengthen at cellular level: Add Frankincense and Helichrysum to the Massage Blend Technique during inflammation phase 2x daily. 2 drops Frankincense to base of neck, rub up towards the base of skull 2x daily. 2 drops Frankincense under tongue morning and night, hold then swallow.

Legend: Preferred, Suggested, Consider

Or 2 capsules or 16 drops of Cellular Complex Blend daily is also suggested for cellular support.

Anxiety and discomfort: Topically apply or diffuse Grounding Blend, Restful Blend or other oils pleasant to the individual.

Pain and stimulation: Topically apply Peppermint, White Fir or Soothing Blend with carrier oil for sensitive skin.

Alzheimer's

Oils: Frankincense[C], Lavender, Melissa[C], Patchouli[C] **Blends/Products:** Basic Vitality Supplements, Focus Blend[C], Grounding Blend, Massage Blend, Restful Blend

Basic health and prevention: Basic Vitality Supplements with 1-3 drops Grounding Blend, Frankincense or Melissa to brain stem 2x daily.

Depression and sleep: Diffuse Restful Blend or Lavender. Massage Blend Technique weekly or more often if possible.

Agitation and depression: 1-2 drops of Melissa and/or Frankincense on brain stem, bottoms of feet, roof of mouth or under the tongue.

Cognitive impairment: 1-2 drops of Focus Blend or Patchouli on brain stem or bottoms of feet or 1-2 drops Patchouli on roof of mouth or under the tongue.

Other oils: Clove[C], Ginger[C], Myrrh[C], Oregano[C], Peppermint, Rosemary, Thyme[C], Vetiver[C], Ylang Ylang[C]

Amenorrhea (absence of menstrual periods)

see also Hormonal balance

Oils: Basil[EC], Clary Sage[EC], Peppermint[EC], Roman Chamomile[EC] **Blends/Products:** Phytoestrogen Complex, Monthly Blend for Women

Phytoestrogen Complex and Monthly Blend for Women are specifically formulated to balance hormones and manage menstrual problems.

The other oils above are also suggested by both early and contemporary experts. Consider cup & inhale and/or use a warm compress after applying oils topically to the abdomen.

Other oils: Lavender[EC], Marjoram[EC], Rosemary[EC], Yarrow[C]

Amnesia · *see* Memory

Amoebic dysentery

Oils: Lavender[C], Lemon, Oregano **Blends:** Digestive Blend, Protective Blend

2-3 drops Lavender in capsule 2x daily or 3-5 drops each Digestive Blend and Protective Blend (or Oregano) to a capsule and take 3x per day. 2-4 weeks may be required. More difficult, use same capsule protocol but a rectal application 2x daily.

Prevention during travel: 2 drops each Lemon and Protective Blend in mouthful of water 1-2x daily.

Other oils: Cinnamon Bark, Melaleuca, Roman Chamomile, Thyme

Note: The common Amoebic Dysentery is a parasitic infection. While we were compiling this information we studied the works of six authors, some foundational and others more contemporary. Anti-parasitic was one of the property classifications we studied. Five oils were cited by at least three of these experts for parasitic infections: Cinnamon Bark, Lemon, Mountain Savory, Oregano, Roman Chamomile.

Analgesic · *see* Pain

Anemia *(iron deficiency)*

Oils: Cinnamon Bark[C], Ginger[C], Grapefruit[C], Lemon[EC] **Blends/Products:** Basic Vitality Supplements

Basic Vitality Supplements with "green smoothie" every day. Simple green smoothie is: 1/4 fresh pineapple, 3 cups baby spinach or kale, 1 drop Peppermint oil, 2-3 cups water blended. Plenty of water and to each 10 oz add: 2 drops each Lemon, Grapefruit, Ginger, Cinnamon Bark.

Other oils: Lavender, Peppermint, Roman Chamomile[E], Thyme[E], Ylang Ylang, Grounding Blend

Aneurysm

Oils: Cypress[C], Frankincense[C], Helichrysum[C]

1-2 drops each Frankincense, Helichrysum and Cypress topically with

Legend: Preferred, Suggested, Consider

light massage 2x daily.

Diffusing and/or the Massage Blend Technique periodically plus Basic Vitality Supplements for foundational health.

Caution: Aneurysm symptoms should be considered potentially life threatening and should have professional medical attention.

Other oils: Clary Sage^C, Melaleuca^C **Blends:** Cellular Complex Blend, Massage Blend, Soothing Blend

Anger   *see* Irritability

Angina   *see also* Heart conditions

Oils: Ginger^C, Peppermint, Wintergreen^C **Blends:** Grounding Blend^C

Grounding Blend and Wintergreen applied topically (dilute with a carrier for those with sensitive skin) directly to the heart area or reflexology points on feet or hands. Alternate with Ginger and Peppermint. Also use inhalation or diffusing.

Other oils: Wild Orange^EC

Angular cheilitis   *see* Chapped lips

Animal bites   *see also* Scar reduction, Snake bites

Oils: Frankincense, Melaleuca **Blends:** Cleansing Blend, Protective Blend

No broken skin: Clean/apply Melaleuca. Soothing Blend for pain.

Puncture wound: Clean/apply Cleansing Blend with carrier topically, work into puncture, cover. Repeat 2x or more times daily for 2-3 days or until process is complete.

Open wounds with torn flesh: Helichrysum and pressure to stop bleeding. Clean/apply Frankincense and Cleansing Blend.

Cautions: If stitches are required or potential damage to ligaments, nerves, etc. seek professional medical attention. If risk of rabies, capture animal if possible and seek professional medical attention.

Infection protection: 4 drops Protective Blend, 3 drops Oregano in capsule, 2x daily.

Other oils: Basil, Clove, Helichrysum, Lavender[E], Oregano **Blends:** Soothing Blend

Animals (pets)

Cats	*see* Cat care
Dogs	*see* Dog care
Horses	*see* Horse care

[*Robert Tisserand (an EO expert) writes that it is safe to use EO in small amounts with cats while others raise more serious concerns. Conclusion: Be very cautious especially with older and sensitive pets.*]

Editorial comment: The following was contributed by an interested essential oil user.

In regards to using essential oils around animals - extreme caution should be taken when birds are involved. Tea Tree (or Melaleuca) oil is extremely toxic to birds (including parrots.) Inhaling, absorbing, or ingesting are all lethal. Pine oils can also be hazardous. Parrots are much more sensitive to inhalants than many other animals. The aromas of the oils can cause distress as well. If you are using oils near a bird, and the bird appears to be in distress, get the bird to fresh air immediately, and consult with your avian veterinarian.

Ankylosing spondylitis
(severe arthritic condition of the back)

Oils: Birch, Marjoram, Peppermint **Blends/Products:** Basic Vitality Supplements, Massage Blend, Soothing Blend, Soothing Blend Rub

Soothing Blend augmented with Birch, Marjoram and Peppermint applied topically. Periodic use of Massage Blend Technique and consistent Basic Vitality Supplements.

Other oils: Basil, Cassia, Eucalyptus, Vetiver

Anorexia

Emotional: Oils: Bergamot, Lavender, Rose **Blends:** Joyful Blend, Restful Blend
Appetite: Oils: Frankincense[C], Grapefruit[C] **Blends:** Invigorating Blend[C]

Legend: Preferred, Suggested, Consider

Emotional: Addressing the mental/emotional dimension is very important. Can be life threatening, seek professional help for serious concerns and use oils to supplement:

    Soothing/calming: Lavender, Restful Blend, Ylang Ylang

    Emotional calm plus appetite help: Bergamot, Invigorating Blend, Frankincense (works for pets as well)

    Self-esteem/self worth: Grounding Blend, Joyful Blend

    Accepting sexuality: Rose, Blend for Women

Diffuse, cup & inhale or warm baths with appropriate oils.

Appetite: 1-3 drops Invigorating Blend (other oils) to each glass water.

Other Emotional: Oils: Ylang Ylang Blends: Blend for Women, Grounding Blend, Invigorating Blend

Other Appetite: Oils: Cardamom[EC], Fennel[E], Roman Chamomile[E], Yarrow[C]

Anosmia   see Smell, loss of

Anti-Aging Blend (immortal skin)

essential oils
Blend

(comes in a roll-on dispenser)

Ingredients: Frankincense, Helichrysum, Lavender, Myrrh, Rose, Sandalwood (Hawaiian)

Addresses: Aging, damage from sun, inflammation, maintain moisture, nourish skin, tissue renewal

(see Safety Chart, page 23)

Antibacterial   see also Bacterial infection

This is a partial list of oils and blends with antibacterial properties:

Basil[C], Cardamom[C], Cinnamon Bark[C], Clove[C], Frankincense[C], Lemon[EC], Lime[C], Melaleuca[C], Protective Blend[C], Cleansing Blend[C], Oregano[C], Spikenard[C], Thyme[EC]

Blue Tansy[C], Cassia[C], Clary Sage[C], Copaiba[C], Cypress[C], Elemi[C], Eucalyptus[C], Geranium[EC], Grapefruit[C], Helichrysum[C], Lavender[C], Jasmine, Lemongrass[C], Marjoram[EC], Myrrh, Neroli[C], Peppermint[C], Ravensara[C], Roman Chamomile[E], Rosemary[EC], Siberian Fir[C], Wild Orange, Respiratory Blend[C], Topical Blend

Antibiotic *(anti-infectious)*

see Bacterial infections, Fungal infections, Viral infections

Antibiotics destroy microorganisms in the body such as bacteria, fungi or parasites. Protective Blend and Protective Blend + are blends of the most effective antibiotic oils. *See also* antibacterial, antifungal and antiviral.

Anticatarrhal   *see* Congestion

Anticoagulant   *see also* Blood clots

This is a partial list of oils and blends with anticoagulant properties:
Grapefruit^C, Helichrysum^C

Clove^C, Cypress^C, Fennel^C, Lemon^C, Lemongrass^C, Thyme^C

Antidepressant   *see* Depression

Antifungal   *see also* Fungal infections

This is a partial list of oils and blends with antifungal properties:
Cinnamon Bark^C, Topical Blend^C, Clove^C, Melaleuca^C, Protective Blend^C, Oregano^C, Rosemary^C, Spikenard^C, Thyme^{EC}

Cassia^C, Cedarwood^C, Clary Sage^C, Copaiba^C, Cypress^C, Elemi^C, Eucalyptus^C, Fennel^C, Geranium^C, Grapefruit^C, Helichrysum^C, Lavender^C, Lemon^C, Lemongrass^C, Marjoram^C, Melissa^C, Myrrh^C, Patchouli^C, Peppermint^C, Ravensara^C, Roman Chamomile^C, Siberian Fir^C, Wild Orange^C, Wintergreen^C

Antihemorrhage   *see* Hemorrhage

Antihistamine   *see* Allergies

Anti-infectious   *see* Antibiotic

Anti-inflammatory   *see* Inflammation

Antimicrobial
see Antiseptic and Disinfectants

Antimicrobial substances destroy microorganisms such as bacteria, fungi or parasites. Antiseptics are antimicrobial substances that are applied to living tissue and disinfectants are antimicrobial substances that are applied to non-living areas to destroy microorganisms.

Antimucolytic
see Congestion

Antioxidant

This is a partial list of oils and blends know for their antioxidant properties:
Clove[C], Douglas Fir[C], White Fir[C]

Cinnamon Bark[C], Copaiba[C], Frankincense[C], Helichrysum[C], Melaleuca[C], Oregano[C], Peppermint[C], Petitgrain[C], Roman Chamomile[C], Rosemary[C], Thyme[C], Cleansing Blend[C], Protective Blend[C], Respiratory Blend[C], Soothing Blend[C], Yarrow-Pomegranate Blend[C]

Antiparasitic
see also Parasite infections

This is a partial list of oils and blends with antiparasitical properties:
Cinnamon Bark[E], Lemon[EC], Melaleuca[C], Oregano[C], Roman Chamomile[EC], Thyme[EC], Cleansing Blend, Digestive Blend[C], GI Cleansing Formula

Bergamot[E], Clove[C], Eucalyptus[E], Fennel[C], Lavender[C], Melissa[E], Neroli[C], Peppermint[EC], Rosemary[C]

Antirheumatic
see Arthritis

Antiseptic
see also Bacterial infections, Fungal infections, Viral infections

Antiseptics are antimicrobial substances that are applied to destroy microorganisms. This is a partial list of oils and blends with antiseptic properties:

Cinnamon Bark[EC], Cleansing Blend, Protective Blend, Protective Blend Foaming Hand Wash

Basil[E], Bergamot[E], Cassia[C], Cedarwood[EC], Clove[E], Douglas Fir[C], Eucalyptus[E], Frankincense[C], Ginger[C], Grapefruit[C], Jasmine[E], Juniper

Berry[EC], Lavender[E], Lemon[C], Lemongrass[C], Myrrh[C], Neroli[E], Ravensara[C], Rosemary[E], Siberian Fir[C], Thyme[E], Wild Orange[C], Yarrow[C], Ylang Ylang[EC]

Antispasmodic

This is a partial list of oils and blends with antispasmodic properties:
Bergamot[E], Black Pepper[E], Cypress[EC], Frankincense, Massage Blend, Soothing Blend

Basil[E], Birch, Cassia, Cilantro, Cinnamon Bark[E], Clary Sage[E], Clove[E], Eucalyptus[E], Fennel[E], Helichrysum, Jasmine, Juniper Berry[EC], Lavender[E], Marjoram[E], Melissa[E], Neroli[EC], Peppermint[E], Petitgrain, Roman Chamomile[E], Rose[E], Rosemary[E], Sandalwood[E], Siberian Fir[C], Thyme, Yarrow[C], Ylang Ylang

Antiviral   *see also* Viral infection

This is a partial list of oils and blends with antiviral properties:
Basil, Cassia, Cinnamon Bark[C], Topical Blend, Clove[C], Eucalyptus[C], Frankincense, Helichrysum[C], Lemon[C], Lemongrass, Marjoram, Melaleuca[C], Melissa[C], Myrrh[C], Oregano[C], Thyme[C], Protective Blend[C], Respiratory Blend[C]

Clary Sage[C], Grapefruit[C], Lime[C], Neroli[C], Peppermint[C], Ravensara[C], Sandalwood[C]

Ants and insects   *see* Household care, Insect repellent

Anxiety *(fear/calming)*

Oils: Frankincense[C], Lavender[C], Melissa[C], Ylang Ylang[C] **Blends/ Products:** Comforting Blend[C], Focus Blend, Grounding Blend[C], Joyful Blend[C], Massage Blend[C], Renewing Blend, Respiratory Blend[C], Restful Blend

Topically apply preferred oil to the chest and/or wrists during the day. Some rotate oils others find one best. Apply Lavender to the bottoms of the feet for improved sleep. For an anxiety attack use cup & inhale for immediate relief. Some suggest Neroli or other oils applied before events that may be stressful can be very helpful. Respiratory Blend is strongly suggested for interrupting anxiety attacks.

Other oils/blends: Bergamot^C, Cedarwood^EC, Copaiba^C, Fortifying Blend^C, Green Mandarin^EC, Jasmine^C, Litsea^EC, Magnolia^C, Manuka^C, Neroli^E, Petitgrain^EC, Pink Pepper^C, Spikenard^EC, Star Anise^C, Tangerine^C, Turmeric^C, Vetiver^C, Yarrow-Pomeranage Blend^C

Apathy   *see* Mood swings

Aphrodisiac   *see also* Erectile dysfunction, Libido

Oils: Rose^EC, Sandalwood^EC, Ylang Ylang^EC **Blends:** Anti-Aging Blend^C, Blend for Women^C

Anti-Aging Blend or blend 3 drops Ylang Ylang with 1 drop Wild Orange or blend Lemongrass, Vetiver and Ylang Ylang. Diffuse or apply topically with roller bottle over thyroid area, behind ears and on wrists.

Other oils: Cardamom^E, Cinnamon Bark^EC, Clary Sage^EC, Cumin^C, Jasmine^EC, Lemongrass, Neroli^EC, Patchouli^E, Star Anise^C, Vetiver, Wild Orange

Appetite

Loss of   *see* Anorexia
Suppressant   *see* Weight loss

Arborvitae *(Thuja plicata)*

essential●oil

Properties: Antibacterial, antiseptic, calming

Addresses: Alopecia, coughs, fevers, psoriasis, rheumatism, skin care, UTI, warts

(see Safety Chart, page 23)

Arrhythmia *(tachycarida)*   *see* Heart conditions

Arteriosclerosis   *see* Heart conditions

Arthritis   *see also* Joint pain, Autoimmune diseases
(Joint stiffness, Osteoarthritis, Rheumatoid arthritis, Rheumatism)

Oils: Birch^C, Copaiba^C, Lavender^EC, Oregano^EC, Peppermint^C, Wintergreen^C **Blends/Products:** Soothing Blend^C, Soothing Blend Rub^C

Temporary pain relief: Apply topically Birch, Soothing Blend (Rub), Frankincense, Peppermint and/or Wintergreen to affected area. Some find Soothing Blend Rub with an added drop of Soothing Blend more effective. Follow with modest warmth from heat pad. Use carrier oil for sensitive skin. Since arthritis is often chronic consider rotating oils.

Long term relief: Consistent Basic Vitality Supplements, weekly Massage Blend Technique and cleansing protocols. Some report very positive results using Copaiba topically consistently.

Other oils: Basil[C], Cassia[C], Cedarwood[C], Cinnamon[C], Douglas Fir[C], Frankincense[C], Ginger[C], Grapefruit[C], Helichrysum[EC], Juniper Berry[E], Lemon[EC], Marjoram[C], Myrrh[C], Pink Pepper[C], Siberian Fir[C], Star Anise[C], Turmeric[C], Yarrow[C], Ylang Ylang[C] **Blends/Products:** Basic Vitality Supplements, Massage Blend

Asperger's   *see* Autism

Asthma

Oils: Cypress[EC], Eucalyptus[EC], Frankincense[EC], Lavender[EC], Rosemary[EC] **Blends/Products:** Respiratory Blend[C]

Each person varies. Normally for immediate easing use topically rather than inhalation. Start with gentle oils like Lavender, then progress to oils with more expectorant properties like Eucalyptus. Use Rosemary for calming.

Prevent attacks: 2-4 drops of Grounding Blend on the bottom of each foot morning and night. Layer Bergamot after Grounding Blend on feet for stress. Diffuse. Take a capsule with 3-5 drops Frankincense 2x daily.

During attacks: 2-4 drops Respiratory Blend on back and chest, augment with Lime or layer with Rosemary.

Mild asthma: Carry Respiratory Blend for exercise-induced asthma.

Other oils: Bergamot, Blue Tansy[EC], Cedarwood[C], Ginger[C], Lemon[EC], Lime, Marjoram[EC], Myrrh[C], Peppermint[C], Thyme[EC], Ylang Ylang[C] **Blends/Products:** Basic Vitality Supplements, Grounding Blend

Astringent   *see also* Hemorrhage

This is a partial list of oils and blends with astringent properties:
Cedarwood[EC], Cinnamon Bark[E], Copaiba[C], Cypress[EC], Douglas Fir[C],
Frankincense[E], Geranium[E], Juniper Berry[EC], Myrrh[E], Neroli, Patchouli[E],
Peppermint[E], Rose[E], Rosemary[E], Sandalwood[E], Yarrow[C]

Atherosclerosis   *see* Heart conditions

Athlete's foot

Oils: Lavender[C], Melaleuca[C], Thyme[C] **Blends/Products:** Protective
Blend[C], Topical Blend[C]

Topical Blend or make blend of equal parts Lavender, Melaleuca, and
Thyme. 2-3 drops of either blend on area of infection 3x daily for 10 days.
Follow with Melaleuca (may be mixed 3:1 with carrier oil) for 30 days to
insure fungus does not return.

Additional itching relief: Lavender topically

Reoccurrence: Consider shoes may be contaminated. Place cotton ball
with Melaleuca or Cleansing Blend in each shoe in bag overnight.

Other oils: Copaiba[C], Cypress[C], Geranium[C], Lemongrass[C], Neroli[C],
Oregano[C]

Atrial fibrillation   *see* Heart conditions

Attention deficit disorder   *see* ADD/ADHD

Auditory processing disorder   *see also* SPD

Oils: Lemon[C], Lime, Vetiver[C] **Blends:** Grounding Blend[C]

Based on very limited experience, diffusion of Wild Orange, Vetiver or
Lime in the classroom was successful.

Other oils: Peppermint

Autism and Asperger's

Oils: Frankincense[C], Lavender[C], Patchouli[C], Vetiver[C] **Blends:** Focus
Blend, Invigorating Blend[C], Restful Blend[C]

[Note: Many with these disorders are very sensitive to odors/touch. Do not force application of oils if it is a negative experience.]

Focus: Focus Blend is a blend specifically prepared to enhance focus and support healthy thought processes. Vetiver (and/or Frankincense) oil carried in a pocket or worn on a clay necklace during the day may support the ability to stay calm and improve focus. Clay necklaces with oil or apply oil to area between thumb and first finger is an easy quick technique to inhale during a busy school day.

Rest: Nightly foot massages or diffusing with Lavender or other relaxing oils. Many find success letting the child choose their own oils.

Diet: Basic Vitality Supplements (reduce quantities depending on age) and test for and eliminate any food or household chemical allergies.

Peaceful Child Blend: Some have had success with the blend known as Peaceful Child applied to bottoms of feet and brain/spinal reflexology points of feet after morning shower.

Other oils: Clary Sage[C], Helichrysum[C], Marjoram, Sandalwood[C], Ylang Ylang **Blends:** Grounding Blend[C], Peaceful Child Blend

Autoimmune diseases

Addison's disease	*see* Adrenal conditions
Celiac disease	*see* Celiac disease
Colitis	*see* Inflammatory bowel disease
Crohn's disease	*see* Crohn's disease
Diabetes type 1	*see* Diabetes
Grave's disease	*see* Thyroid conditions
Hashimoto's thyroiditis	*see* Thyroid conditions
Infla..tory Bowel Disease (IBD)	*see* Inflammatory bowel disease
Lupus	*see* Lupus
Multiple sclerosis	*see* Multiple sclerosis
Narcolepsy	*see* Narcolepsy
Rheumatoid arthritis	*see* Arthritis
Schmidt's syndrome	*see* Adrenal conditions
Scleroderma	*see* Scleroderma
Sjogren's syndrome	*see* Sjogren's syndrome
Ulcerative colitis	*see* Inflammatory bowel disease

Oils: Frankincense **Blends/Products:** Basic Vitality Supplements, Cellular Complex Blend, GI Cleansing Formula/Probiotic Defense Formula

Legend: Preferred, Suggested, Consider

Nutrition: Basic Vitality Supplements consistently, Cellular Complex Blend 8 drops or 1 capsule 2x daily.

Support: 2-3 drops Frankincense 2-4x daily.

Symptoms and protection: Use oils for specific symptoms and protection from contagious disease.

Emotional support: Use Grounding Blend, Invigorating Blend, Joyful Blend, Lavender, etc.

Organ cleanse: Detoxification Blend protocol, see Detoxification.

Candida cleanse: Some suggest a root cause of autoimmune diseases is Candida and may be addressed with a gastrointestinal cleanse, see Detoxification.

Notes:

Legend: Preferred, Suggested, Consider

Babies   *see* Infant care

Back conditions

Bone spurs   *see* Bone spurs
Osteoarthritis   *see* Arthritis
Sciatica   *see* Sciatica

[Back pain, Disk degeneration, Failed back syndrome, Herniated disc, Lumbago, Neck pain, Spina bifida, Spinal stenosis, Whiplash]

Oils: Cypress^C, Frankincense, Helichrysum^C, Myrrh^C **Blends/Products:** Massage Blend, Soothing Blend, Soothing Blend Rub

Use at least daily. Remember back pain needs to be addressed at multiple levels, supplement the Massage Blend Technique with these:

Immediate pain relief:· Soothing Blend or Soothing Blend Rub (or Birch or Wintergreen). 2-3 drops topically to area of pain as needed.

Reduce inflammation: Myrrh (or Bergamot, Black Pepper, Roman Chamomile or Rosemary). 2-3 drops topically where nerve is being pinched 2-3x daily.

Relax muscles/spasms: Massage Blend (or Lavender, Lime, Marjoram or Melissa). 2-3 drops to area where spasm is occurring.

Increase circulation: Cypress (or Invigorating Blend, Eucalyptus, Geranium, Lemon or Peppermint). 2-3 drops to spinal area 2-3x per day.

Encourage additional help and tissue regeneration: Helichrysum (and Frankincense or Sandalwood). 1-2 drops topically to spinal area 2-3x per day followed by a hot compress.

Other oils: Bergamot^E, Birch, Black Pepper^E, Invigorating Blend^C, Eucalyptus^C, Geranium^C, Lemon^C, Lime^C, Marjoram^C, Peppermint^C, Roman Chamomile^{EC}, Sandalwood^C, Thyme^{EC}, Wintergreen^C

Bacterial infections

Oils: Basil[C], Cardamom[C], Cinnamon Bark[C], Clove[C], Coriander[C], Eucalyptus[C], Geranium[EC], Oregano[C], Rosemary[EC], Thyme[EC] **Blends:** Protective Blend[C]

The oils above are scientifically proven antibacterial agents. Because some oils are more effective against different strains of bacteria than others consider a blend for unknown bacteria. See the individual health concerns (Cuts and wounds, Food poisoning, etc) for application techniques. The suggested oils below are also noted by some to be effective antibacterial agents. Most essential oils have antibacterial properties. Go to antibacterial for many other oils.

Other oils: Bergamot[C], Copaiba[C], Grapefruit[C], Green Mandarin[C], Lemon[EC], Lemongrass[C], Lime[C], Manuka[C], Wild Orange[C] **Blends:** Cleansing Blend[C]

Bad breath (halitosis)

Oils: Cardamom[EC], Peppermint[EC] **Blends/Products:** Digestive Blend, Peppermint Beadlets, Protective Blend

Breath freshener: 2 Peppermint Beadlets, swallow one then let other one dissolve in mouth; or put 2 drops of Peppermint directly in mouth.

Oral bacteria is source: Oil pulling with Protective Blend or Peppermint after brushing and/or tongue scraping.

Digestive tract is source: 1-2 drops of Digestive Blend after each meal.

Other oils: Bergamot[E], Cilantro[C], Cinnamon Bark[C], Cumin[C], Dill[C], Lavender[EC], Lemongrass[C], Patchouli[C], Spearmint[C], Thyme[C]

Bags under eyes

Oils: Cypress, Frankincense **Products:** Tightening Serum

Root cause: Water retention (see edema), lack of sleep (see insomnia).

Daily: Cypress blended with Frankincense (or oils below) and VCO at night, Cypress neat in mornings.

Other oils: Geranium, Myrrh, Sandalwood **Products:** Anti-Aging Moisturizer (*see* Skin care)

Balance *see Vertigo*

Baldness *(alopecia, hair loss)*

Oils: Clary Sage[C], Cypress[C], Lavender[EC], Rosemary[EC] **Blends/Products:** Basic Vitality Supplements[C], Salon Essentials Protecting Shampoo, Smoothing Conditioner and Root to Tip Serum

Use Salon Essentials Protecting Shampoo and Smoothing Conditioner, Basic Vitality Supplements to build strong hair. Consider supplementing the Essential Oil Hair Serum and/or with oils below plus using oils/blends for hormonal balance if needed.

Mild hair loss: Add 1-2 drops of Rosemary to shampoo daily.

Serious hair loss: Shampoo daily with these oils added to shampoo: 3 drops Rosemary, 5 drops Lavender, 4 drops Cypress, 4 drops Clary Sage. Use Basic Vitality Supplements consistently.

Other oils: Arborvitae[C], Lemon[C], Roman Chamomile[C], Spikenard, Thyme[EC], Wintergreen[C], Yarrow[C], Ylang Ylang[C]

Basal cell carcinoma *see Skin cancer*

Basic Vitality Supplements

Product

see also Supplements, Children's supplements

Basic Vitality Supplements mentioned often in this book are an important part of many suggestions. These are also available as vegan products. Most often it is recommended that a three part regiment of such supplements be used:

Cellular Vitality Supplements: Food nutrients with bioavailable vitamins and minerals that are commonly deficient in our modern diets.

Essential Oil Omega Complex: Marine and land-sourced omega fatty acids. Can include Clove and other essential oils and is available in vegan friendly formulation.

Food Nutrient Complex: A source of natural botanical extracts that can support healthy cell proliferation, lifespan and energy.

Also note that these same nutritional benefits are available in products for children and others that may have swallowing difficulties. See Children's supplements.

Basil *(Ocimum basilicum)*

essential oil

Properties: Antibiotic, antidepressant, anti-inflammatory, antiseptic, decongestant, disinfectant, expectorant

Addresses: Bronchitis. cold and flu, depression, earache, migraine, insect bites, stress

(see Safety Chart, page 23)

Bed bugs

Oils: Lemongrass **Blends:** Cleansing Blend[C]

To remove from area: In spray bottle mix 1/4 cup water with 15 drops Lemongrass or Clove/Peppermint. Strip bed, spray mattress (carpets if suspected). Wash bed linens, add small towel with 3-5 drops Cleansing Blend to dryer. Spray sheets and pillow cases daily for 3-5 days. Also diffuse above oils for 2-4 hours with mattress uncovered and closet doors open.

For relief from bites: Cleansing Blend (or Lavender, Repellent Blend) applied topically to area.

Other oils: Clove, Lavender[EC], Peppermint **Blends:** Outdoor Blend, Protective Blend

Bedsores *(pressure ulcers)*

Oils: Helichrysum, Frankincense[C], Lavender[C], Melaleuca[C], Rosemary **Products:** Basic Vitality Supplements

2-5 drops (depending on area) Helichrysum/Lavender or Melaleuca/Rosemary to area 3x daily. Add Frankincense to hasten results. Basic Vitality Supplements for system support.

Other oils: Cypress, Geranium, Marjoram, Myrrh, Ylang Ylang

Legend: Preferred, Suggested, Consider

Bedwetting

Oils: Cilantro, Cypress[EC], Rosemary[EC] **Blends:** Grounding Blend

Experiment since there are many root causes.

7 drops Cilantro in capsule 2x daily, 2-4 drops Cypress on bladder area before sleep, 2-4 drops Grounding Blend on feet at bedtime with massage and quality, loving, reinforcing time. Rub diuretic oils such as Rosemary on the feet and ankles 2 -3 hours before bedtime.

Some suggest Basic Vitality Supplements and GI Cleansing Formula/ Probiotic Defense Formula

Other oils: Copaiba[C], Grapefruit[C], Lemon[C] **Blends/Products:** Basic Vitality Supplements, GI Cleansing Formula/Probiotic Defense Formula

Bee stings

[including Wasps, Yellow Jackets]

Oils: Basil[C] **Blends:** Cleansing Blend[C], Protective Blend[C]

Some simple suggestions are:

> For bees and others that may leave the stinging mechanism (stinger) in the skin gently rub over the area with a fingernail or such to remove this source of infection.

> Lightly wash the area with soap (Protective Blend foaming wash is excellent) and water.

> **Dab 2-3 drops Basil** or any of the recommended oils **directly on area bitten as soon as possible**. Repeat if necessary every 1 or 2 hours.

> For young children or very sensitive skin dilute oils with a carrier.

> Avoid scratching as much as possible.

Special Precautions: For severe reactions or a considerable number of bites or stings, consult a professional healthcare specialist. (Some folks that have severe allergic reactions should be prepared with an anaphylaxis kit.)

Other oils: Cinnamon Bark[C], Lavender[C] **Blends:** Repellent Blend[C]

Bell's palsy
see also Nerve damage

Oils: Frankincense, Helichrysum **Blends:** Protective Blend

Viral infection (most common root cause): 3-5 drops Protective Blend in capsule 2-3x daily.

Encourage repair of facial nerve: 2-3 drops Frankincense and/or Helichrysum topically below ear and to affected area of the face.

Other oils: Oregano, Peppermint^C, Rosemary^C, Thyme^C

Benign prostatic hypertrophy
see Prostate conditions

Bergamot *(Citrus bergamia)*

essential oil

Properties: Analgesic, antibiotic, antidepressant, anti-inflammatory, antiseptic, antispasmodic, antiparasitic, astringent, digestive, sedative

Addresses: Anxiety, depression, eczema, indigestion, insomnia, psoriasis, stress, urinary tract infection

(see Safety Chart, page 23)

Bipolar *(manic depression)*

Oils: Frankincense^C, Melissa **Blends/Products:** Basic Vitality Supplements, Grounding Blend^C, Joyful Blend, Restful Blend^C

Proper nutritional balance: Healthy eating and Basic Vitality Supplements.

Clarify/focus: Inhale Grounding Blend (Frankincense or Vetiver). Carry Grounding Blend at all times, apply to wrists, back of neck and/or inhale.

Lift/energize: Joyful Blend topically and/or inhale.

Stress relief: Melissa on upper lip and back of neck. Also inhalation of Lavender. Use these oils with foot massage.

Rest and sleep: Restful Blend diffused or the bottom of the feet.

Other oils: Clary Sage^C, Lavender^C, Vetiver^C **Blends:** Invigorating Blend^C

Legend: Preferred, Suggested, Consider

Birch *(Betula lenta)*

essential oil

Properties: Analgesic, anti-inflammatory, antiseptic, antispasmodic, disinfectant, diuretic, stimulant, sedative

Addresses: Arthritis, bone spurs, cramps, deodorant, diuretic, eczema, gout, hypertension, joint pain, muscle pain, psoriasis, skin toner, tendonitis

(see Safety Chart, page 23)

Bird flusee Flu

Birdssee Animals

Birthingsee Childbirth

Bites

Animals	*see* Animal bites
Insects	*see* Insect bites
Snakes	*see* Snake bites

Black Pepper *(Piper nigrum)*

essential oil

Properties: Anti-inflammatory, antiseptic, circulatory, diuretic, stimulant

Addresses: Arthritis, bruising, constipation, immune strengthener, indigestion, joint pain, muscle pain, poor circulation

(see Safety Chart, page 23)

Bladder cancersee Cancer

Bladder infectionsee UTI

Bladder wall inflammation *(interstitial cystitis)*   *see also* UTI

Oils: Frankincense

Some recommend an organic tampon with 6-8 drops of Frankincense inserted over night. Repeat until symptoms improve. Also Basic Vitality Supplements coupled with proper diet.

Bleeding   *see* Hemorrhage

Bleeding during pregnancy   *see* Pregnancy

Blend

Definition When individual essential oils are combined together the resulting "combination of oils" is referred to as a blend. The blend usually combines oils that are complementary to each other and work together. Commercial companies often prepare blends and give them unique and sometimes trademarked names. These blends can also be identified by a generic description that gives a succinct phrase that captures how the blend might help.

In this book we describe 29 blends and use these generic terms. Anti-Aging Blend, Blend for Women, Calming Blend (old name), Cellular Complex, Cleansing Blend, Detoxification Blend, Digestive Blend, Focus Blend, Grounding Blend, Invigorating Blend, Joyful Blend, Massage Blend, Metabolic Blend, Monthly Blend for Women, Outdoor Blend (new name), Protective Blend, Protective Blend+, Repellent Blend (old name), Respiratory Blend, Restful Blend (new name), Seasonal Blend, Soothing Blend, Tension Blend, Topical Blend.

Blend for Women *(whispers gentle soothing relief)*

essential oils
Blend

Ingredients: Bergamot, Cinnamon Bark, Cocoa bean absolute, Jasmine flower absolute, Labdanum, Patchouli, Rose, Sandalwood (Hawaiian), Vanilla bean absolute, Vetiver, Ylang Ylang in a base of Fractionated Coconut Oil

Another common formulation: Clary Sage, Geranium,

Legend: Preferred, Suggested, Consider

Idaho Tansy, Jasmine, Lavender, Orange, Rosewood, Sage, Sandalwood, Vetiver, Ylang Ylang

Addresses: An all natural compelling fragrance that contains no synthetic toxic chemicals. Wonderful for women and a great cologne for men.

(see Safety Chart, page 23)

Blisters   see also Cuts and wounds

Oils: Lavender[C], Melaleuca[C] **Blends:** Protective Blend

Clean area with Protective Blend. Drain blister with disinfected needle (Protective Blend). Apply Lavender (Melaleuca or Myrrh) topically every 1-2 hours.

Other oils: Copaiba[C], Geranium[C], Helichrysum[C], Myrrh[C] **Blends:** Cleansing Blend[C]

Bloating

[aerophagy (bloating from swallowing air)]

Oils: Lemon[E], Peppermint[C] **Blends/Products:** Basic Vitality Supplements, Digestive Blend, Digestive Enzyme Complex, Metabolic Blend

Immediate relief: Digestive Blend or blend of Lemon, Peppermint, Rosemary on tummy area or 3-5 drops Digestive Blend in capsule.

Chronic bloating: Basic Vitality Supplements consistently, 1-3 Digestive Enzyme Complex capsules with meals. Also recommended is Metabolic Blend before meals (capsules starting at 3 drops each, increase to max 8).

Prevention: 1-3 capsules Digestive Enzyme Complex prior to or with the meals that may cause problems.

Other oils: Coriander[E], Fennel[E], Marjoram[E], Oregano[E], Rosemary **Blends/Products:** GI Cleansing Formula, Probiotic Defense Formula

Blood clots   see also Anticoagulant

[Deep vein thrombosis (DVT)]

Oils: Cypress[C], Helichrysum[C] **Blends/Products:** Basic Vitality Supplements, Massage Blend, Soothing Blend

Ongoing: Consistently use Basic Vitality Supplements, drink lots of water.

DVT: Blood clots in major blood vessels can be life threatening. Seek professional medical attention. Complementary help with essential oils can be considered as described under superficial phlebitis below.

Superficial phlebitis (and DVT after clots are addressed):

If painful: Pat or spray (do not massage or rub directly) Massage Blend, Soothing Blend Rub or Peppermint.

Additional help: 2-3 drops each Cypress and Helichrysum to bottoms of feet 2-3 times daily. If area is not painful Cypress and Helichrysum can be applied directly to area, follow with hot compress.

Note: The doseage for pharmaceutical medications for DVT are usually monitored and regulated carefully. Simultaneous use of anticoagulant essential oils can alter the optimum levels of the pharmaceuticals and their use should be coordinated with the attending medical professional. Some find Helichrysum initially gives a tingling or painful feeling as it helps. This sensation is temporary and will go away.

Other oils: Clove, Fennel[C], Grapefruit[C], Lemon[C], Lemongrass[C], Thyme[C]
Blends: Grounding Blend

Blood conditions

Blood clots	*see* Blood clots
Bloody nose	*see* Nosebleed
Cholesterol	*see* Cholesterol control
Deep vein thrombosis (DVT)	*see* Blood clots
Hemorrhage (bleeding)	*see* Hemorrhage
High blood pressure	*see* Hypertension
Low blood pressure	*see* Hypotension

Blue Tansy *(Tanacetum annum)*　　　also know as Moroccan Chamomile

Properties: Analgesic, antibacterial, antihistamine, anti-inflammatory, calming, cooling

Addresses: Anxiety, asthma, emphysema, irritability, itchy skin, mood swings, muscle pain, muscle stiffness, radiation damage, seasonal allergies, stress, sunburn

　　Legend: Preferred, Suggested, Consider

Special note: Be sure that you are obtaining an oil that is specifically distilled from Tanacetum annuum. Tansy (Tanacetum vulgare) and Blue Tansy (Tanacetum annuum) oils are very different oils.

(see Safety Chart, page 23)

Body lotions   see Personal care and Skin care

Body odor   see also Deodorant (natural) and Personal care
[Excess perspiration, Foot odor, Underarm odor]

Oils: Bergamot[E], Cypress[EC], Lemongrass **Blends:** Cleansing Blend[C], Natural Deodorant

Different oils will blend best with different bodies and any underlying health conditions. Apply oils directly or premix oils with a carrier oil in a 1-5% dilution (3-15 drops to 1 Tbsp of carrier oil).

Also consider a ready-made deodorant products made from essential oils like Natural Deodorant made with Cypress, Melaleuca, Cedarwood and Bergamot.

For excess perspiration consider Cypress, Litsea or Petitgrain.

Other oils: Black Pepper[E], Cedarwood, Cilantro[C], Clary Sage[E], Eucalyptus[E], Frankincense[E], Geranium, Litsea[C], Manuka[C], Melaleuca, Neroli[EC], Patchouli[E], Peppermint, Petitgrain[C], Siberian Fir[C], Spikenard[C] **Blends:** Blend for Women[C], Invigorating Blend, Joyful Blend[C], Restful Blend[C]

Boils (and carbuncles)

Oils: Frankincense[C], Lavender[EC], Oregano, Rosemary, Thyme[C]

4 drops each Oregano, Rosemary and Thyme in a capsule internally 3x daily until gone. For the sores apply 1-2 drops each Lavender and Frankincense directly to soothe, then Helichrysum after sore is closed to regenerate and minimize scarring.

Other oils: Clary Sage[EC], Lemon[EC], Melaleuca[C] **Blends:** Cleansing Blend[C]

Bone cancer   see Cancer

Bone Nutrient Complex *(Women's bone support supplement)*

essential oils
Product

The Bone Nutrient Complex is a blend of vitamins and minerals that are essential for bone health including vitamins C and D, calcium, magnesium and other trace minerals. It can be used by women (and men) of all ages as a dietary supplement to conveniently increase consumption of the bone nutrients found in healthy foods but often deficient in our modern diets.

Bone spurs

Oils: Cypress[C], Eucalyptus, Frankincense, Helichrysum, Marjoram[C], Peppermint, Thyme, Wintergreen[C] **Blends/Products:** Massage Blend, Soothing Blend

Pain relief: Soothing Blend or Wintergreen topically to area or use the Massage Blend Technique.

Additional help: Blend 4 drops each Cypress, Eucalyptus, Frankincense, Helichrysum, Marjoram, Peppermint, Wintergreen with 10 drops coconut oil. Apply blend to affected area 2x daily until bone spur is gone, continue thereafter for 2 weeks. Accelerate results by wrapping with warm cloth after oils applied, then wrap with plastic bag and additional towel.

An alternative blend: 5 drops each Eucalyptus, Marjoram, Cypress, Lavender, Thyme, Basil with 30 drops coconut oil.

Other oils: Lavender[C], Thyme

Bone, broken *(fracture)*

Pain:

> **Oils:** Wintergreen **Blends:** Soothing Blend, Soothing Blend Rub
>
> Topically apply to injured area Soothing Blend, Soothing Blend Rub or Wintergreen as needed.

Additional help:

> **Oils:** Birch, Cypress, Helichrysum, Lemongrass, Marjoram, White Fir
>
> Topically apply Cypress, Helichrysum (most important) and White Fir to the injured area 2 to 3 times a day. If there is ligament or

Legend: Preferred, Suggested, Consider

tendon damage add Lemongrass. If there is muscle damage add Marjoram.

Calming:
Oils: Lavender **Blends:** Grounding Blend

Diffuse or cup & inhale Grounding Blend and/or Lavender.

Improve nutrition:
Blends/Products: Basic Vitality Supplements, Bone Nutrient Complex

Other oils: Clove, Eucalyptus, Ginger, Oregano, Vetiver

Botulism	*see* Food poisoning

Bowel obstruction	*see* Constipation

BPH *(benign prostatic hypertrophy)*	*see* Prostate conditions

Brain cancer	*see* Cancer

Breast cancer	*see* Cancer

Breastfeeding *(lactation, nursing)*	*see also* Childbirth, Pregnancy

Basic cautions

Some report decreased milk supply with Peppermint, others do not. To err on the side of caution Peppermint and blends using Peppermint (Digestive Blend, Metabolic Blend) should be limited if milk production is at risk. Be aware this summary does not include all cautions one should be aware of and we advise reading the cautions for any oil recommended. See Safety Considerations section at the beginning of this book.

Some point out: 1) What mothers ingest is passed through to breast milk so "hot" oils or certain tastes may effect some infants, 2) Toxins eliminated during detoxification can be passed to breast milk.

Breast engorgement
see Decreasing milk supply below

Decreasing milk supply

Oils: Peppermint

3-5 drops of Peppermint to cup warm water with honey and drink or 3-5 drops topically with a carrier oil.

Other blend: Blend for Women[C]

Increasing milk supply

Oils: Clary Sage[C], Fennel[EC], Geranium[E]

15 drops Fennel or Geranium or 10 drops Clary Sage to 2 Tbsp carrier oil. Topically to breasts and surrounding areas 1x daily. Drink lots of water, relax and be patient.

Other oils: Jasmine, Lemongrass[E]

Mastitis

Oils: Basil, Frankincense **Blends:** Protective Blend

1-3 drops each Frankincense, Protective Blend and Basil, rub on affected area and bottoms of feet. Repeat every hour first day and every 2 hours second day. Be aggressive and consistent.

Also 2-4 drops each Frankincense and Protective Blend in capsule every 2 hours.

Other oils: Lavender[C] **Blends:** Invigorating Blend[C]

Sore nipples

Oils: Lavender, Helichrysum, Roman Chamomile[C]

Use snug nursing bra with nursing cups. Also, after nursing apply Lavender, Helichrysum or Roman Chamomile mixed with carrier oil.

Breast tumors   *see* Tumors

see also   Abscess, Cysts, Lipoma, Polyps

Broken bone   *see* Bone, broken

Bronchitis

Oils: Basil, Cypress[C], Eucalyptus[EC], Frankincense, Lemon[E], Rosemary[E]

Legend: Preferred, Suggested, Consider

Blends: Protective Blend, Respiratory Blend

2-4 drops Respiratory Blend topically to chest for coughing (supplement with Eucalyptus or Rosemary). 1-3 drops Protective Blend (dilute for some) topically on throat as antibiotic (supplement with Basil, Frankincense or Lemon). For severe bronchitis 1-3 drops Protective Blend in capsule 2-4x daily.

Also diffuse Respiratory Blend (Eucalyptus or Rosemary) or cup & inhale.

Other oils: Cedarwood[E], Douglas Fir[C], Elemi[C], Lavender[EC], Manuka[C], Oregano[EC], Peppermint[C], Ravensara[C], Siberian Fir[C], Thyme[E]

Bruise (contusion, hematoma)

Oils: Cypress[C], Geranium[C], Helichrysum[C], Lavender[C], Lemongrass[C]
Blends/Products: Soothing Blend[C]

Immediately: Apply Lavender or Soothing Blend for pain and Helichrysum and/or Cypress to constrict blood vessels, increase vessel constriction with cold compress, repeat every 1-2 hours.

After 6-24 hours: Apply blend of 5 drops Helichrysum, 3 drops each Cypress, Geranium, Lavender and Lemongrass to area 2-3x daily. Alternate hot and cold compresses to speed process.

Other oils: Fennel[EC], Myrrh[C], Rosemary[C]

Bug bites   see Insect bites

Bulimia   see Anorexia

Bulimia, as with anorexia, is an eating disorder that is accompanied by emotional/mental challenges. The steps suggested under anorexia might provide the foundation for dealing with bulimia.

Bunions

Oils: Cypress[C], Lemongrass[C], Wintergreen **Blends:** Massage Blend

Apply Lemongrass with Massage Blend and Wintergreen to the area for pain and help. Follow oils with warm washcloth, plastic bag, towel or sock for 1-2 hours. Also consider 2-5 drops Lemongrass on bottoms of feet and back of neck at least 2x daily.

Results vary from a few weeks to months. Cypress improves circulation and Basic Vitality Supplements encourages the process.

Other blends: Anti-Aging Blend, Grounding Blend, Respiratory Blend, Soothing Blend, Tension Blend

Burns   *see also* Scar reduction

Oils: Frankincense[C], Helichrysum[C], Lavender[EC], Melaleuca[C], Peppermint[C], White Fir[C]

Immediate: Cover area with Frankincense or Lavender neat, follow with Peppermint to cool. For large areas or sensitivity make a spritz.

Blistering: Apply Melaleuca or Frankincense to prevent infection.

Pain: Apply White Fir, this also prevents infection.

Scarring: Apply Helichrysum.

Radiation: 3 d Helichrysum, 2 d Blue Tansy with carrier oil applied topically.

Other oils: Blue Tansy[E], Copaiba[C], Geranium[EC], Marjoram **Blends:** Protective Blend[C]

Bursitis

Oils: Cypress[C], Lemongrass, Marjoram[C], Wintergreen[C] **Blends:** Soothing Blend[C]

Apply combinations of above oils 3x daily until the pain is reduced, then taper off.

Pain and inflammation: Soothing Blend or Wintergreen

Circulation: Cypress

Additional help: Lemongrass or Marjoram

Other oils: Basil[C], Birch, Ginger[C], White Fir[C] **Blends:** Tension Blend

Notes:

_____

_____

_____

Legend: Preferred, Suggested, Consider

Calluses (and Corns)

Oils: Grapefruit[C], Oregano[C] **Blends:** Topical Blend[C]

2-3 drops of one of the oils topically to corn or callus area at least 2x daily. Continue consistently until softened, then remove.

Other oils: Clove[C], Lemon[C], Myrrh[C], Peppermint[C], Roman Chamomile[C]

Calming   see Anxiety

Calming Blend   see Restful Blend

Campylobacter enteritis   see Food poisoning

Cancer   see also Skin cancer
[Bladder, Bone, Brain, Breast, Cervical, Colon, Esophageal, Hodgkin disease, Leukemia, Liver, Lung, Ovarian, Prostate, Stomach, Throat, Testicular, Uterine, ...]

Oils: Clove[EC], Frankincense[C], Lavender[C], Sandalwood[C], Thyme[C]

Cancer conditions, as with many other serious health issues, should have treatment that includes professional medical attention.

Ongoing research has shown Frankincense effective in reducing cancerous tumors. Clove, Lavender, Sandalwood and Thyme are also oils found to be anti-tumoral. Other research findings include Patchouli for cervical, Myrtle for breast and prostate, Grapefruit for skin cancer. Many oils are also helpful for pain, radiation burns (see Burns) and support tissue regeneration.

Consider medical professional doctors who also recognize the benefits of complementary natural approaches.

Prevention: 2 drops Frankincense under the tongue daily.

Candida (yeast infection)   see also Thrush, Vaginitis

Oils: Lemon[EC], Melaleuca[C], Oregano[C], Spikenard[C] **Blends/Products:** GI Cleansing Formula/Probiotic Defense Formula

Children (18 months to 5 years): GI Cleansing Formula/Probiotic Defense Formula protocol adapted for children. Break open 1 GI Cleansing Formula capsule, apply to bottoms of feet 2x daily with meals. Dab for small children, proportionally more for older children, continue 7-10 days. Follow with 1 or 2 Probiotic Defense Formula capsules (depending on age) internally daily for 5 days. For those that cannot take capsules the best alternative is to break open the Probiotic Defense Formula capsules and mix with applesauce.

Adults: GI Cleansing Formula/Probiotic Defense Formula cleanse: 1-3 GI Cleansing Formula capsules daily with meals for 10 days, follow with Probiotic Defense Formula, 3 capsules per day with meals for 5 days. Repeat monthly if necessary.

Similar cleanse: 5 drops Lemon and Melaleuca with 3 drops Oregano in capsule. Take 2x daily, 10-14 days, rest 2 weeks, repeat.

Discomfort: *see* Vaginitis

Other oils: Lavender^C, Myrrh^{EC}, Neroli^C, Rosemary^C **Blends/Products:** Detoxification Blend

Candidiasis
see Candida

Canker sores

Oils: Frankincense, Myrrh^{EC} **Blends:** Protective Blend^C

1-2 drops topically directly on the canker sore. It usually requires 1-2 applications. Protective Blend may need to be diluted with a carrier oil, especially for children.

Other oils: Lemon, Lemongrass, Melaleuca^C

Capsules
see also Conversions, Diluting, Drops

Definition Empty capsules (veggie as well) may be purchased (at health food stores, etc) and used for taking oils internally.

Capsule size	# of mg	# of drops
00 capsule	735	15-20
0 capsule	500	10-13

Legend: Preferred, Suggested, Consider

Car sick
see Motion sickness

Carbuncles
see Boils

Cardamom *(Elettaria cardamomum)*

essential oil **Properties:** Antibiotic, antiseptic, antispasmodic, aphrodisiac, digestive, diuretic, stimulant

Addresses: Acid reflux, appetite (loss of), colic, cough, dyspepsia, flatulence, halitosis, headaches, sciatica, vomiting

Cardiomyopathy
see Heart conditions

Cardiovascular conditions
see Heart conditions

Carpal tunnel

Oils: Cypress[C], Helichrysum, Lemongrass[C] **Blends:** Massage Blend[C], Soothing Blend[C]

Pain: Topically apply Birch, Soothing Blend (Rub) or Wintergreen to wrist as needed.

Additional help: 1-2 drops Massage Blend or Cypress (circulation), Frankincense or Helichrysum (nerve damage), Lemongrass (connective tissue) and Marjoram (muscle tissue) 2-3x daily.

Other oils: Basil[C], Frankincense[C], Marjoram, Oregano[C], White Fir, Wintergreen

Carrier oil
see also Lotions

Definition A mild, light oil that may be used to mix with an essential oil for those with sensitive skin and/or to assist in massaging oils into the skin. Common carrier oils are Coconut Oil (FCO - fractionated coconut oil, VCO - virgin coconut oil, EVCO - extra virgin coconut oil), Grapeseed Oil, Jojoba Oil, Olive Oil, Safflower Oil. Mixing an essential oil with a carrier does not decrease the effectiveness of the essential oil.

Cartilage injury
see Knee injury

Cassia *(Cinnamomum casssia)*

Properties: Antibiotic, antidiarrhea, antiseptic, antispasmodic, antiviral, astringent, disinfectant, stimulant

Addresses: Arthritic pain, cold and flu, constipation, cough, diarrhea, stomachache

(see Safety Chart, page 23)

Cat care

Oils: Lavender, Melaleuca^C **Blends:** Restful Blend

[Robert Tisserand (an EO expert) writes that it is safe to use EO in small amounts with cats while others raise more serious concerns. Conclusion: Be very cautious especially with older and sensitive pets. Also be wary of citrus and pine oils that are not of high quality.]

Cuts and wounds: 1-2 drops essential oil diluted with FCO on wound.

Ear mites: A report suggests 3% Melaleuca in olive oil.

Soothe: 1-2 drops Restful Blend on hands, let kitty inhale to soothe during travel and grooming visits.

Cataracts   *see* Eyesight failing

Catarrh   *see* Congestion

Cavities   *see* Teeth conditions

Cedarwood *(Juniperus virginiana)*

Properties: Analgesic, astringent, calming, insect repellent, sedative

Addresses: Acne, anxiety, dandruff, eczema, psoriasis and other skin disorders, skin care, wounds

(see Safety Chart, page 23)

Celiac disease   *see also* Autoimmune diseases

Oils: Grapefruit[C], Ginger[C], Lemon[C] **Blends/Products:** Basic Vitality Supplements, Cellular Complex Blend[C], Digestive Enzyme Complex[C], GI Cleansing Formula

These seem common to successes: Avoid gluten; cleanse and re-establish healthful bacteria using GI Cleansing Formula/Probiotic Defense Formula, use Digestive Enzyme Complex for improved digestive function, consistently use Basic Vitality Supplements, drink sufficient pure water; avoid sodas/caffeine.

For ongoing support: Basic Vitality Supplements, 2 drops each Lemon, Grapefruit, Ginger, with 1 drop Cinnamon Bark in a capsule 1-3x daily.

Enhance nutrition with Green Smoothies to add more iron.

Other oils: Cinnamon Bark[C], Frankincense, Melaleuca[C], Oregano[C], Peppermint **Blends/Products:** Digestive Blend

Cellular Complex Blend *(key ingredients for cellular health)*

essential oils (also available in Softgels)
Blend

Ingredients: Clove, Frankincense, Lemongrass, Niaouli leaf, Summer Savory plant, Thyme, Wild Orange

Addresses: Cellular health, cellular apoptosis, cellular renewal, protects DNA from free-radical damage, provides antioxidants

(see Safety Chart, page 23)

Cellular Complex Blend Softgels

essential oils   The same as the Cellular Complex Blend with 8 drops of the
Product   blend in a single easy to swallow softgel.

Cellulite reduction

Oils: Helichrysum[C] **Blends/Products:** Metabolic Blend[C], Metabolic Blend Trim Shakes

Topically apply Helichrysum essential oil then layer with Metabolic Blend on locations with cellulite and other fatty accumulations.

Couple with full Metabolic Blend protocol as described under weight loss if necessary.

Other oils: Cumin[C], Cypress[EC], Grapefruit[C], Lime[C], Oregano[EC], Tangerine[C], Wild Orange[C]

Cellulitis

Oils: Frankincense, Melaleuca, Oregano **Blends/Products:** Anti-Aging Blend, Protective Blend

4 drops each Frankincense, Melaleuca, Protective Blend, Oregano in a capsule 3x daily and topically on the infected area.

For orbital or periorbital cellulites dot Anti-Aging Blend around eye socket 3x daily.

Other oils: Lavender[E], Rosemary[E], Spikenard, Yarrow[C] **Blends/Products:** GI Cleansing Formula/Probiotic Defense Formula, Topical Blend

Centering Blend (a Yoga blend)

essential oils
Blend

Ingredients: Bergamot Fruit, Coriander Seed, Marjoram Leaf, Peppermint, Geranium, Basil, Rose, Jasmine Flower

Addresses: Brings a new sense of peace and purpose, leading to a renewal of resolution and direction.

(see Safety Chart, page 23)

Cerebral palsy

Oils: Clary Sage[C], Frankincense[C], Helichrysum[C], Peppermint **Blends/Products:** Grounding Blend, Massage Blend, Respiratory Blend[C] and the additional oils/blends used in the Massage Blend Technique: Soothing Blend, Lavender, Melaleuca, Protective Blend and Wild Orange

---

Legend: Preferred, Suggested, Consider

Primarily: The Massage Blend Technique daily to weekly is most recommended.

Augment: Grounding Blend, Frankincense and/or Helichrysum along spine followed with Peppermint then light massage.

Breathing difficulties: Use Respiratory Blend with cup & inhale, topically to chest or diffusion.

Other oils: Basil, Clary Sage, Roman Chamomile

Cervical cancer   see Cancer

CFS   see Chronic Fatigue Syndrome

Chamomile, Moroccan   see Blue Tansy

Chamomile, Roman   see Roman Chamomile

Change, dealing with   see Emotional strength

Chapped lips (angular cheilitis)   see also Lip balm

Oils: Frankincense, Lavender[C] **Blends/Products:** Basic Vitality Supplements, Lip Balm (Herbal), Lip Balm (Tropical), Lip Balm (Wild Orange and Peppermint)

The Lip Balm with Essential Oils or 15 drops each Frankincense and Lavender with 1 Tbsp carrier oil in roller bottle, apply frequently to the affected area. Drink lots of water, Basic Vitality Supplements for the essential fatty acids.

Other oils: Geranium[C], Lemon[C], Melaleuca[C], Sandalwood

Chapped skin   see also Skin care, infants

Oils: Geranium[C], Jasmine[C], Lavender, Myrrh[C], Spikenard[C] **Blends/Products:** Anti-Aging Moisturizer, Hydrating Cream (*see* Skin care), Protective Blend, VCO

Apply Anti-Aging Moisturizer and/or Hydrating Cream to affected area. Also Myrrh neat or in an ointment of 12-30 drops Myrhh and 1 ounce Virgin Coconut Oil.

Root cause may be dietary. Consistently use Basic Vitality Supplements.

Other oils: Clary Sage, Copaiba[C], Elemi[C], Helichrysum, Magnolia[C], Neroli[EC], Roman Chamomile[E], Wintergreen

Chapstick
see Lip balm

Charlie horse
see Muscle cramps

Chemical constituents

Definition In some descriptions of essential oils a list of chemical constituents of the oil will be given. There are a number of reason this may be important to you.

1) Essential oils with common chemical constituents will often have similar properties and may help you find an alternative if needed.

2) The knowledge of chemical constituents is often used to determine which oils will blend together effectively.

3) The chemical composition of an oil is what is tested to determine both its purity and often its potency. It should be noted that there may well be some constituents that are very high in an oil (ie 50% to 80%) but a beneficial trait of an oil may well come from a minor constituent or a combination of particular consituents. Here are some common constituents found in essential oils and their major beneficial characteristics:

HYDROCARBONS

Terpenes (monoterpenes, sesquiterpenes, limonene, pinene) vary greatly but include antibacterial, antiseptic, antiviral.

  Monoterpenes (Grapefruit, Lemon, Orange)

  Susquiterpenes (in most oils but high percentage in Cedarwood, Ginger, Myrrh, Patchouli, Roman Chamomile, Rose, Sandalwood)

Legend: Preferred, Suggested, Consider

OXYGENATED COMPOUNDS

Aldehydes may be calming when inhaled, anti-infectious, anti-inflammatory but may be skin sensitive (Cinnamon Bark, Lemon, Lemongrass, Melissa, Myrrh)

Alcohols

> **Monoterpene alcohols** are usually antiseptic, antifungal, antiviral (Geranium, Juniper, Lavender, Melaleuca, Rose)

> **Sesquiterpene alcohols** may have anti-inflammatory or benefit allergies (Patchouli, Sandalwood, Vetiver)

Esters typically are very aromatic and are often found to be relaxing and antifungal, antispasmodic (Bergamot, Clary Sage, Lavender, Petitgrain, Roman Chamomile)

Ketones are beneficial for mucus and upper respiratory conditions but also toxic in some instances (Rosemary)

Oxides (1,8-cineol or eucalyptol) may be anesthetic, antiseptic and an effective expectorant (Eucalyptus)

Phenols (eugenol, thymol, carvacrol) may be antiseptic, antibacterial, disinfectant but the oil may also be "hot" or possible irritating to the skin. (Cinnamon Bark, Clove, Oregano, Thyme)

Chewable Multivitamins *see* Children's supplements

Chickenpox

Oils: Lavender[C], Lemon[C], Melaleuca[C] **Blends/Products:** Protective Blend

Local itching: 3 drops each Lavender and Melaleuca with each oz of Calamine lotion, apply topically.

Extensive areas: 1 cup baking soda with 2-4 drops Lavender to warm bath. Mix well, let small child soak and play.

Avoid spreading: Diffuse Protective Blend or 2-3 drops Protective Blend in capsule for others in contact.

Flu-like symptoms: 2-3 drops Lemon oil and honey in cup of warm water.

Other oils: Bergamot[C], Eucalyptus[C], Frankincense, Geranium, Lemongrass, Roman Chamomile[C], Thyme

Chiggers

Oils: Lavender[C], Melaleuca[C] **Blends:** Cellular Complex Blend

Some simple suggestions are:

> Lightly wash the area with soap (Protective Blend foaming wash is excellent) and water.

> Dab 2-3 drops of Melaleuca or any of the recommended oils directly on areas bitten as soon as possible.

> Repeat if necessary every 1 or 2 hours.

> For young children or very sensitive skin dilute oils with a carrier.

> Avoid scratching as much as possible.

Other oils: Lemongrass, Thyme **Blends/Products:** Repellent Blend

Chilblains   *see also* Frostbite

Oils: Helichrysum, Lavender, Myrrh

Apply Lavender to relieve discomfort. Topical application of Myrrh and Helichrysum will aid in repairing blood vessels and surrounding tissue.

Other oils: Geranium, Lemon[E], Melaleuca

Childbirth   *see also* Breastfeeding, Pregnancy

see also the book *Essential Oils for Pregnancy, Birth & Babies* by Stephanie Fritz LM, CPM.

Delivery

Baby position
Myrrh[C], Peppermint[C]
Myrrh and/or Peppermint with FCO applied to abdomen may help turn a baby who is breach.

Calming during early labor
Clary Sage[C], Geranium[C], Lavender[C], Grounding Blend[C], Massage Blend[C]

Legend: Preferred, Suggested, Consider

Apply single or blend of above with FCO to back and shoulders or undiluted on bottoms of the feet.

Labor
Slowing early labor: Lavender[c]
1-3 drops Lavender applied to abdomen.

More effective contractions: Clary Sage[c], Geranium[c], Lavender[c]
Clary Sage with Geranium or Lavender applied to inside of ankles, bottoms of feet, lower abdomen and lower back.

Intensify and move along: Clary Sage[c], Myrrh[c]
Myrrh or Clary Sage with Myrrh applied to inside of ankles, bottoms of feet, lower abdomen and lower back.

For pain: Basil[c], Black Pepper[c]
Basil or Black Pepper with FCO massaged on lower back.

Labor room atmosphere
Lavender[c], Wild Orange[c], Grounding Blend[c], Invigorating Blend[c]

Diffuse lightly Lavender, Invigorating Blend, Grounding Blend or Wild Orange. Be certain aroma is soothing to new mom.

Perineum care
Before delivery: Clary Sage[c], Frankincense[c], Geranium[c], Helichrysum[c], Lavender[c], Rose[c]
Make spray of 8 drops Geranium, 5 drops Lavender and 1 oz FCO and apply 2-3x daily the week prior to delivery.

During delivery: Frankincense[c], Helichrysum[c]
5 drops each Helichrysum, Frankincense with 1 Tbsp FCO, gently massaged on perineum during crowning and on baby's head during birth.

Post Delivery

After pains
Massage Blend[c], Monthly Blend for Women[c], Soothing Blend[c], Lavender[c]

1-3 drops Massage Blend, Soothing Blend, Lavender or Monthly Blend for Women applied directly to lower abdomen.

Anointing newborn
Frankincense[C]

Many suggest a single drop of Frankincense be applied to the new child's crown and down their spine.

Breastfeeding (lactation, nursing)   *see* Breastfeeding

Caesarean, prevent scarring
Helichrysum[C], Anti-Aging Blend[C], Lavender[C]

Anti-Aging Blend or Helichrysum/Lavender to area to promote help and prevent scarring. Apply topically, at least daily, until improvement is visible.

Circumcision
Frankincense[C], Anti-Aging Blend[C], Lavender[C]

Anti-Aging Blend or Frankincense/Lavender with FCO applied directly for help.

Hemorrhoids
Cypress[C], Helichrysum[C], Lavender[C]

1-2 drops each Helichrysum and/or Lavender topically directly to area of discomfort. Add Cypress with carrier if more severe. 2-3 drops in Sitz baths.

Jaundice
Geranium[C], Lemon[C]

1 drop each Geranium and Lemon to bottoms of baby's feet every 3-4 hours.

Perineum care and helping episiotomies
Frankincense[C], Anti-Aging Blend[C], Lavender[C]

2-4 drops Anti-Aging Blend or Frankincense/Lavender with FCO, apply directly or in water spray 3-4x daily.

Postpartum depression
Grounding Blend[C], Clary Sage[C], Frankincense[C], Rose[C], Ylang Ylang[C]; also mentioned are Bergamot[C], Monthly Blend for Women[C], Joyful Blend[C], Geranium[C], Grapefruit[C], Lavender[C], Lemon[C], Myrrh[C],

Sandalwood[C], Wild Orange[C]

Grounding Blend or blend of equal parts Geranium, Lavender, Sandalwood, Ylang Ylang. Diffuse, 2-3 drops to bottoms of feet, 1-2 drops on pillowcase or 5-6 drops in warm bath.

Umbilical cord
Frankincense[C], Myrrh[C]

1 drop Myrrh on stump, continue daily with 1-2 drops Frankincense until cord stump falls off.

Childbirth fever   *see* Pregnancy

Children's Blends *(blends helpful to children)*   *see* Kid's Blends

Children's supplements
see also Supplements, Basic Vitality Supplements

Product Available nutritional supplements for children and others with swallowing difficulties that cannot take capsules include:

Chewable vitamins: These are flavored multivitamins that may include B vitamins with a blend of vitamins A, C, E with botanical extracts.

Omega-3 Fish Oil: Available in liquid form with Wild Orange essential oil flavor to take out the fish taste.

Probiotic: Available in a powdered form.

These will support healthy cell development and longevity when taken daily.

Chills   *see* Fever

Cholecystitis   *see* Gall bladder inflammation

Cholesterol control   *see also* Heart conditions

Oils: Cassia, Lavender[C], Lemongrass[C]

Basic Vitality Supplements a must. Also consider 5-7 drops Lemongrass or 3 drops Lemongrass with 2 drops Cassia or Lavender in capsule daily.

Also use adequate water daily.

Other oils: Basil[C], Helichrysum[E], Rosemary[EC]

Chronic bronchitis   *see* Bronchitis

Chronic fatigue syndrome (CFS)

Oils: Frankincense, Oregano[E], Peppermint[C], Thyme[E] **Blends/Products:** Basic Vitality Supplements[C], GI Cleansing Formula/Probiotic Defense Formula, Protective Blend[C]

GI Cleansing Formula/Probiotic Defense Formula cleansing protocol (*see* Detoxification); raw fruits and vegetables, green smoothies; avoid sugars, processed foods, dairy. Basic Vitality Supplements consistently. Use Protective Blend, Oregano and/or Thyme internally in a capsule for candida and other infections, Frankincense for helping, Peppermint for invigoration.

Other oils: Basil[C], Blue Tansy[C], Cinnamon Bark[E], Clove[E], Lemongrass[C], Wild Orange, Melaleuca[E] **Blends:** Digestive Blend[C]

Chronic inflammation   *see* Inflammation

Chronic obstructive pulmonary disease   *see* COPD

Cigarettes   *see* Addictions

Cilantro (Coriandrum sativum)

 essential oil

Properties: Analgesic, antibacterial, antifungal, antioxidant, antispasmodic, digestive stimulant

Addresses: Arthritis, colds, colic, diarrhea, exhaustion, flatulence, flu, indigestion, migraines, muscle pain, nausea, rheumatism

(see Safety Chart, page 23)

Cinnamon Bark *(Cinnamomum zeylanicum)*

Properties: Antibiotic, antidiarrhea, antiseptic, antispasmodic, antiviral, astringent, disinfectant, stimulant

Addresses: Cold and flu, constipation, cough, diarrhea, insect bites, stomachache

(see Safety Chart, page 23)

Circulation, poor   *see also* Heart conditions

Oils: Cypress^C, Frankincense^C, Lemongrass, Marjoram^C **Blends/Products:** Basic Vitality Supplements, Massage Blend, Protective Blend

Long term: Basic Vitality Supplements

Short term relief for mild symptoms: Add Massage Blend, Cypress or Protective Blend to Hand & Body Lotion or VCO and massage on feet and vigorously on the insides of calves and/or forearms, always towards heart.

Relief for difficult symptoms: Use the above massage application of oils plus blend equal parts Cypress, Marjoram, Lemongrass, Frankincense and rub onto chest near heart and the bottoms of feet.

Neuropathy protocol helps some: Rub 2-4 drops Grounding Blend on the feet, rub 2-4 drops each of Basil, Cypress and Marjoram on one foot, then 2-4 drops Peppermint, cover with hot towel. Repeat on other foot.

Other: Black Pepper^C, Coriander^C, Green Mandarin^{EC}, Lemon^{EC}, Rosemary^{EC}, Thyme^{EC} **Blends/Products:** Invigorating Blend^C

Cirrhosis   *see* Liver conditions

Clary Sage *(Salvia sclarea)*

Properties: Antibacterial, antidepressant, antifungal, anti-inflammatory, antiseptic, antispasmodic, astringent, hormone stimulant

Addresses: Acne, circulation, dandruff, depression, frigidity, gastric spasms, hair loss, hormone balance, hot flashes, hypertension, impotence, menopause, migraines/headaches, painful menstruation, PMS, whooping cough, wrinkles

(see Safety Chart, page 23)

Cleaning, household *see* Household care

Cleansing Blend *(a purifying blend)*

Blend

Ingredients: Austrian Fir needle, Cilantro, Citronella grass, Lemon, Lime, Melaleuca, Pine needle, Siberian Fir needle

Another common formulation: Citronella, Lavandin, Lemongrass, Melaleuca, Myrtle, Rosemary

Addresses: Cuts and wounds, disinfects surfaces, insect bites, kills airborne pathogens, supports immune system

(see Safety Chart, page 23)

Cleansing, body internal *see* Detoxification

Cleansing, body topical *see* Personal care

Cleansing, facial topical *see* Skin care

Clove *(Eugenia caryophyllata)*

essential oil

Properties: Analgesic, antibiotic, antidepressant, anti-inflammatory, antiseptic, disinfectant, diuretic, sedative

Addresses: Acne, cold and flu, constipation, cuts and wounds, earache, gum problems, headaches, insect bites, insect repellent, nausea, skin care, toothache

(see Safety Chart, page 23)

Cockroaches *see* Insect repellent

Cognitive impairment *see* Mental acuity

Legend: Preferred, Suggested, Consider

Cold sores *(Herpes simplex, HHV-1)*

Oils: Lemongrass[C], Melaleuca[C], Melissa[C]

1-2 drops Melissa or Lemongrass to outbreak area every 2 hours (not less than 3 times per day). Continue for 3 days after symptoms are gone. For small children 50/50 dilution with a carrier oil.

Additional protection: 1-2 drops Melissa in capsule 3x daily.

Strengthen immune system and emotions: Massage Blend Technique.

Reduce toxins: GI Cleansing Formula/Probiotic Defense Formula and/or Detoxification Blend cleansing.

Other oils: Frankincense[C]/Sandalwood[C] or Lavender[EC], Lemon[EC], Peppermint[C], **Blends/Products:** Detoxification Blend, GI Cleansing Formula/Probiotic Defense Formula, Massage Blend, Protective Blend[C]

Colds

Oils: Cypress[C], Eucalyptus[EC], Lemon[EC], Melaleuca[C], Oregano[C], Peppermint[EC], Rosemary[EC], Thyme[EC] **Blends/Products:** Cleansing Blend[C], Protective Blend[C], Respiratory Blend[C]

Antiviral: Oregano (a "hot" oil, always dilute), Protective Blend, Melaleuca, Frankincense

Remember numerous oils are antiviral. 2-4 drops to feet or chest, throat or internally by gargling or capsule. For internal use with children (not infants) 3/4 tsp honey with 1-2 drops of the chosen oil. Use oils at the first signs. Infants apply diluted (not Oregano) to bottoms of feet.

Fever: Peppermint, Eucalyptus topically to forehead, chest or feet.

Nasal congestion: Respiratory Blend, Lavender/Lemon/Peppermint inhaled via a diffuser or cup & inhale.

Cough and chest congestion: Cypress, Eucalyptus, Lime, Melaleuca or Peppermint applied topically to chest, steam tent and/or with lymph massage.

Other oils: Cinnamon Bark[EC], Frankincense[C], Lavender[C], Lime[C], Manuka[C], Ravensara[C] **Blends:** Invigorating Blend

Colic

Oils: Ginger^C, Lavender^EC, Peppermint^EC **Blends:** Digestive Blend

Apply a Tbsp of carrier oil on the tummy followed by 1-2 drops of Digestive Blend (or one of the other listed oils). Warm hands, massage baby's tummy and lower back with circular motions. Hold and cuddle baby close afterwards. Apply a warm compress after the massage and place on stomach or back. Applying essential oil/carrier oil mixture to feet with a foot massage is also effective.

Other oils: Bergamot^EC, Black Pepper^EC, Cardamom^EC, Coriander^C, Cumin^C, Fennel^E, Geranium^C, Marjoram^EC, Melissa^EC, Neroli^EC, Roman Chamomile^EC

Colitis   *see* Inflammatory bowel disease

Colon cancer   *see* Cancer

Coma   *see* Head injuries

Comforting Blend

essential◐oils
Blend
(comes in a roll-on dispenser)

Ingredients: Amyris, Frankincense, Labdanum, Osmanthus, Patchouli, Rose, Sandalwood, Ylang Ylang

Addresses: An emotional health blend to balance and console during difficult times.

(see Safety Chart, page 23)

Common cold   *see* Colds

Concentration   *see* Mental acuity

Concussion   *see* Head injuries

Conditioner, hair   *see* Hair care

Confusion   *see* Mental acuity

Legend: Preferred, Suggested, Consider

Congenital heart disease   *see* Heart conditions

Congestion

Oils: Eucalyptus[C], Lavender[C], Lemon[C], Lime[C], Peppermint[C] **Blends:** Respiratory Blend[C], Seasonal Blend[C]

Topical: 2-4 drops Respiratory Blend around nostrils and/or on chest. Couple with Eucalyptus for more severe congestion.

Swish and swallow: Seasonal Blend or 2 drops each Lemon, Lavender, Peppermint (more Peppermint for stronger decongestant) in mouthful water. Swish in mouth 20-30 sec, swallow. Repeat every 2-4 hours.

Internal: If too sensitive to swish and swallow take same oils in capsule every 2-4 hours (or Seasonal Blend).

Inhale: Use Respiratory Blend and/or Eucalyptus via diffuser or inhaler; Respiratory Blend from oil bottle, steam tent or cup & inhale.

Other oils: Cedarwood[C], Cinnamon Bark[C], Copaiba[C], Douglas Fir[C], Elemi[C], Lime, Melaleuca[C], Oregano, Siberian Fir[C], Yarrow[C] **Blends:** Protective Blend

Congestive heart failure   *see* Heart condition

Conjunctivitis *(pink eye)*

Oils: Eucalyptus[C], Lavender[EC], Melaleuca[C] **Blends:** Cleansing Blend

Older children/adults: 2-3 drops each Lavender and Melaleuca around socket of eye by putting oils in hand, apply with finger tip.

Younger children: Use hard shell eye patch (pharmacy) with 2 drops each Lavender and Melaleuca to 1/3 of cotton pad placed in patch with oils side of away from eye. Place over affected eye 15-30 minutes, 2-4x daily.

1-2 drops Cleansing Blend on reflexology points. At night apply Eucalyptus (diluted) instead of Cleansing Blend. Repeat daily until redness disappears and two days following.

Caution children not to rub eyes and with small children place socks on feet so oils are not accidentally transferred to eyes. If oils accidentally get in eyes dilute with FCO or another carrier oil, <u>not</u> water.

Other oils: Cypress[C], Frankincense[C], Jasmine[C], Oregano, Spikenard

Constipation

Oils: Black Pepper[E], Cassia[C], Marjoram[EC], Rosemary[EC] **Blends:** Digestive Blend[C], Digestive Enzyme Complex

2-5 drops Digestive Blend neat orally or in capsule.

Also consider: 2 drops each Marjoram and Rosemary with 4 drops carrier oil in capsule or massaged on abdomen.

Infants and children: Use appropriate oils; with infants dilute and rub on bottoms of feet, with children dilute and rub on tummy.

Adults only, heavy duty: 1-5 drops Cassia in cup warm water, drink avoiding lips, add 1 Tbsp honey if preferred. Caution: Cassia is a "hot" oil and should not be used with those that have sensitivities.

Other oils: Cardamom, Dill[C], Fennel[EC], Ginger[C], Lemon[C], Peppermint[C], Rose[EC] **Blends/Products:** Basic Vitallity Supplements, Detoxification Blend

Note: When choosing alternative oils from the list of "**Other oils:**" please review safety precautions on pages 23-28

Contusion
see Bruise

Conversions
see also Capsules, Diluting, Drops

Definition

How many drops are in common containers?

Container	Drops (average)
1 ml	20
5 ml bottle is same as 1 teaspoon	85 (minimum) 100 (average)

Legend: Preferred, Suggested, Consider

Container	Drops (average)
15 ml bottle is same as 1 Tablespoon	250 (minimum) 300 (average)
1 oz	600

Copaiba *(Copaifera reticulata)*

essential oil

(also comes in softgels)

Properties: Analgesic, antibacterial, antifungal, anti-infectious, anti-inflammatory, antimicrobial, antioxidant, antitumoral, astringent, calming, cooling, decongestant, disinfectant, diuretic, mucolytic

Addresses: Acne, arthritis, bacterial infections, calming, cuts & wounds (cuts, disinfect, promote healing, scrapes), emotional conditions (anxiety-fear), fungal infections, high blood pressure, incontinence, joint pain, pain killer, scar reduction, skin care (dry skin, mature skin, wrinkles), stress (tension)

(see Safety Chart, page 23)

COPD *(chronic obstructive pulmonary disease)*   *see also* Cough

Oils: Eucalyptus[E], Lemon[E] **Blends:** Grounding Blend, Respiratory Blend

To help open airways, 3-5 drops Respiratory Blend (or Eucalyptus) diffused and/or applied topically to chest, between nose and upper lip or on hands to cup and breathe at sleep time. 1-2 drops Grounding Blend on feet as well. During day drink water with 1-2 drops Lemon or Wild Orange per glass. Basic Vitality Supplements will also help.

Chronic cough: *See also* Cough

Other oils: Cinnamon Bark, Frankincense, Peppermint[C], Wild Orange

Coriander *(Coriandrum sativum)*

essential oil

Properties: Analgesic, antibacterial, antifungal, anti-inflammatory, antioxidant, antispasmodic, sedative, stimulant

Addresses: Anorexia, flatulence, indigestion, menstrual pain, muscular pain, nausea, stomach spasms, stress

Corns
see Calluses

Corneal ulcer
see Eyesight, failing

Coronary artery spasm
see Heart conditions

Coronary heart disease
see Heart conditions

Cough

Cough: Eucalyptus[EC], Frankincense[EC], Lemon[C], Peppermint[EC], Rosemary[C], Respiratory Blend[C]
Mucus: Lemon[C], Peppermint[EC], Invigorating Blend
Infection: Melaleuca[C], Oregano, Protective Blend[C]

Gargle: 1-2 drops of chosen oil(s) in an ounce of water. Swallow after gargling (some prefer to spit out after gargling).

Cinnamon Bark (STRONG) and lemon (mild)
Protective Blend (strong)
Lavender, Lemon, Peppermint
mild 2,2,2 drops
strong 2,2,4 drops
Oregano (VERY STRONG, may be too strong for some.)

Inhale: Use chosen oils with diffuser, an inhaler, directlly from bottle, make steam tent or cup & inhale.

Topically: Eucalyptus, Melaleuca, Peppermint and/or Cypress to chest and throat areas. Cover with warm compress. (Skin test all but Melaleuca)

Other oils: Basil[C], Cypress[EC], Elemi[C], Green Mandarin[EC], Helicrysum[C], Jasmine[EC], Melissa[C], Myrrh[EC], Ravensara[C], Sandalwood[EC], Star Anise[C], Thyme[C]

Legend: Preferred, Suggested, Consider

Note: When choosing alternative oils from the list of "**Other oils:**" please review safety precautions on pages 23-28.

Courage   *see* Emotional strength

Courage Blend for Children   *see* Kid's Blends

Coxsackievirus A16   *see* Hand-Foot-Mouth disease

Cracked heels *(heel fissures)*

Oils: Melaleuca^C, Peppermint

2-3 drops Melaleuca or Peppermint with VCO, FCO or Hand & Body Lotion topically on area 2x daily, cover with socks. Be consistent and patient.

Another lotion to apply 2x daily. 10 drops each Geranium, Melaleuca, Peppermint blended with VCO, FCO or Hand & Body Lotion.

Other oils: Geranium

Cradle cap

Oils: Geranium^C, Lavender, Melaleuca

1 drop Lavender (or Melaleuca or Geranium) with 1/2 tsp carrier oil, apply to scalp. Let oils absorb into skin before washing the head. After bath apply very small amount of EVCO instead of lotion. 3-4 applications typically needed. Continue for 3-4 days if needed.

Precautions for babies: Skin test first time for any sensitivity.

Other oils: Lemon^C **Blends:** Grounding Blend

Cramps

Menstrual cramps	*see* Dysmenorrhoea
Muscle cramps	*see* Muscle cramps
Stomach cramps	*see* Stomachache

Crohn's disease   *see also* Autoimmune diseases

Oils: Ginger **Blends/Products:** Digestive Blend^C, Probiotic Defense Formula

For at least 6 months take Probiotic Defense Formula 3x daily, 2-4 drops Digestive Blend topically over stomach 2x daily and 2-4 drops Digestive Blend and Ginger on bottoms of feet daily. Important to drink 1/2 of body weight in ounces of water daily (Example: 150 lbs, 75 oz water).

Other oils: Frankincense, Peppermint[C]

Croup
see also Cough

Oils: Frankincense[EC], Peppermint[EC] **Blends:** Respiratory Blend[C]

2 drops each Respiratory Blend, Frankincense and Peppermint to chest with 6-12 drops FCO. Added help apply to bottoms of feet and back. For children dilute with more FCO and for infants only on the bottoms of feet.

Repeat every 1 to 3 hours until coughing stops. Protect small children from transferring oils to their eyes.

Other oils: Lemon[C], Marjoram[EC], Thyme[C]

Cumin *(Cuminum cyminum)*

essential oil

Properties: Antibacterial, antioxidant, antiparasitic, antiseptic, antispasmodic, antiviral, aphrodisiac, digestive

Addresses: Aphrodisaic, bad breath, calming, cellulite reduction, colic, constipation, detoxification, diarrhea, digestive cramps, emotional fatigue or exhaustion, flatulence, headache, indigestion, migraine, muscle cramps, stomachache

(see Safety Chart, page 23)

Cup & inhale

Definition An excellent way to quickly inhale an essential oil or blend. Put a few drops of oils in the palms of the hands, rub them together and cup over the mouth and nose and breathe deeply. For a child do the same with your hands, then cup a single hand near the mouth and nose of the child while they breathe deeply.

Cushing's syndrome
see Adrenal conditions

Legend: Preferred, Suggested, Consider

Cuts and wounds   *see also* Blisters, Scar reduction, Scrapes, Splinters

Oils: Frankincense^EC, Helichrysum^EC, Lavender^EC, Melaleuca^EC **Blends:** Essential Ointment, Protective Blend^C

Minor wounds: Apply Essential Ointment or Lavender neat topically.

More serious wounds:

> **Stopping bleeding:** Helichrysum or Lemon and apply pressure.
>
> **Cleansing:** Protective Blend Foaming Hand Wash is best, Essential Ointment, Protective Blend or Melaleuca oil with soap and water is good.
>
> **Antibiotic:** Essential Ointment, Lavender, Frankincense or Myrrh.
>
> **Pain relief, calming:** Apply Lavender neat to the wound, rub palms together with 2-3 drops of oil and let child inhale the calming fragrance.
>
> **Ongoing:** Repeat application of antibiotic oil every 4-6 hours. Yarrow, Blue Tansy and Copaiba are mentioned to promote healing in wounds. Apply Helichrysum during process to address scarring.

Other oils: Blue Tansy^E, Copaiba^C, Elemi^C, Geranium^EC, Juniper Berry^EC, Lemon^C, Manuka^C, Myrrh^EC, Yarrow

Cypress *(Cupressus sempervirens)*

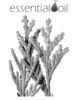

essential oil

Properties: Antibacterial, antibiotic, antiseptic, antispasmodic, astringent, disinfectant, diuretic, sedative

Addresses: Arthritic pain, asthma, cold and flu, diarrhea, excess perspiration, hemorrhoids, insect repellent, menopause, menstrual problems, muscle pain, skin care, sore throat, stress, varicose veins

(see Safety Chart, page 23)

Cystic fibrosis

Oils: Cypress, Eucalyptus, Frankincense, Melaleuca, Peppermint **Blends:** Protective Blend

Nighttime: Diffuse nightly equal parts Eucalyptus and Melaleuca.

2x daily: Massage chest, throat and back using 3 drops each Cypress, Eucalyptus, Frankincense, Melaleuca and 10 drops FCO. After 1 week substitute blend with Respiratory Blend for 3 days then return to the blend. Repeat. Reduce frequency as symptoms diminish.

Added protection: Protective Blend and Peppermint on feet every morning, Respiratory Blend on feet every night and cover with socks.

Emergency attack: Deep inhalation of Respiratory Blend.

Other oils: Geranium, Lavender[c]

Cystitis   *see* UTI

Cysts   *see also* Ganglion cyst, Ovarian cyst, Sebaceous cyst, Tumors

General: Frankincense[c]

Near skin surface: 1-2 drops of Frankincense (or diluted Oregano) topically 2-3x daily until cyst is diminished.

Internal cysts: 1-2 drops Frankincense under tongue 2-3x daily.

Pain from cyst pressure: Soothing Blend or Soothing Blend Rub topically.

Other oils: Basil[c], Lemongrass, Melaleuca, Myrrh, Oregano **Blends:** Soothing Blend

Notes:

_____

_____

_____

_____

_____

Legend: Preferred, Suggested, Consider

Dandruff
see also Hair care

Oils: Lavender[C], Lemon[E], Melaleuca[C], Rosemary[C] **Blends/Products:** Blend for Women, Salon Essentials Protecting Shampoo and Smoothing Conditioner

Light dandruff: Add 2-3 drops Melaleuca or Blend for Women to Salon Essentials Protecting Shampoo or other quality shampoo daily.

Heavy dandruff: Massage 4 drops each Lavender, Lemon, Melaleuca, Rosemary with 1 tsp VCO into scalp nightly. Cover with shower cap, shampoo out next morning.

Other oils: Basil[C], Manuka[C], Roman Chamomile[E], Spikenard, Thyme[C] **Blends/Products:** Basic Vitality Supplements

Decongestant
see also Congestion

This is a partial list of oils and blends with decongesting properties:

Eucalyptus[C], Lime[C], Melaleuca[C], Respiratory Blend, Rosemary[C], Thyme[C], White Fir[C]

Basil, Copaiba[C], Elemi[C], Myrrh, Patchouli, Lavender/Lemon/Peppermint

Deep vein thrombosis (DVT)
see Blood clots

Dehydration
see Heat exhaustion

Delivery at pregnancy
see Pregnancy

Dementia

Oils: Melissa[C], Patchouli[C] **Blends:** Grounding Blend, Massage Blend, Restful Blend

Health and Protection: Basic Vitality Supplements with 1-3 drops Grounding Blend, Frankincense or Melissa topically to brain stem 2x daily.

Depression and sleep: Diffuse Restful Blend or Lavender. The Massage

Blend Technique weekly or more often.

For agitation and depression: 1-2 drops Melissa and/or Frankincense on brain stem or bottoms of feet.

Cognitive impairment: 1-2 drops Patchouli on brain stem or bottoms of feet.

Other oils: Frankincense[C], Geranium[C], Lavender[C], Rosemary[C], Ylang Ylang

Dental conditions

Bad breath	*see* Bad breath
Gum conditions	*see* Gum conditions
Oral hygiene	*see* Oral hygiene
Teeth conditions	*see* Teeth conditions
Teeth grinding	*see* Teeth grinding

Deodorant   *see* Body odor, Deodorant (natural) and Personal care

Deodorant *(natural)*   *see also* Personal care

Ingredients: One suggestion is Bergamot, Cedarwood, Cypress, Meleleuca with an appropriate carrier. Also available commerially with natural additives for smooth application.

Addresses: Body odor.

Caution: Some may be skin sensitive to these oils, discontinue if irritation occurs.

(see Safety Chart, page 23)

Deodorizing areas   *see also* Air quality

Oils: Clary Sage[C], Lemon[C], Peppermint[C], Protective Blend **Blends:** Cleansing Blend[C], Invigorating Blend, Joyful Blend, Restful Blend

Almost all essential oils can be used to enhance the aroma in living spaces. The fragrance chosen is mostly a matter of personal taste. Many oils also have the other benefits spoken of elsewhere in this book. A diffuser is the most straightforward way to enjoy the aromatic benefits. In a car, home or office a tissue with a few drops of an oil may be placed in a vent or in front of a fan. Oil dispensers that heat the oil are not recommended since the high temperature destroys the efficacy of the oils.

Depression

Oils: Bergamot[EC], Frankincense[C], Lavender[EC], Peppermint[C], Wild Orange[C], Ylang Ylang[EC] **Blends/Products:** Basic Vitality Supplements, Grounding Blend, Joyful Blend[C], Restful Blend[C]

Mild depression: Lavender, Neroli, Sandalwood and Ylang Ylang among others. Also Grounding Blend, Joyful Blend and Restful Blend.

Noted expert blend: 2-3 drops each Melissa, Peppermint, Wild Orange.

Diffusion is most effective, but topical application to the chest or body and foot massages or baths also offer good results. For "on the go" use an inhaler or diffusing necklace. Single blends can get "boring" therefore change periodically. Basic Vitality Supplements used consistently.

Other oils: Blue Tansy, Clary Sage[EC], Grapefruit[C], Jasmine[EC], Lemon[EC], Lemongrass[C], Lime[C], Melissa[EC], Marjoram[C], Neroli[EC], Patchouli[EC], Petitgrain[C], Roman Chamomile[EC], Rosemary[C], Sandalwood[EC], Spikenard[C], Tangerine[C] **Blends/Products:** Encouraging Blend, Invigorating Blend[C], Reassuring Blend

Dermatitis
see Eczema

Despair
see Depression

Detoxification

Organ cleansing: Detoxification Blend[C]; Detoxification Complex[C]

Gastrointestinal: GI Cleansing Formula/Probiotic Defense Formula

Two types of basic cleanses:

Nutritional Cleanses: Daily, gentle detoxification can be used indefinitely if necessary.

Organ cleansing (liver, kidneys, colon, lungs and skin): 1 capsule Detoxification Complex 2x daily, morning, evening plus 5 drops Detoxification Blend in a capsule 1x daily or 4 drops each Clove, Geranium, Grapefruit, Rosemary in a capsule 1x daily.

1-3 drops Lemon with each glass of water daily.

Isolated Cleanses: More aggressive, for limited time periods that may address specific parts of the body.

Gastrointestinal tract: GI Cleansing Formula, 3 capsules daily with meals for 10 days (adjust number for age and sensitivity). Follow with Probiotic Defense Formula, 3 capsules daily with meals for 5 days. Rest 10-15 days, repeat 2x if necessary.

There are many other cleanses described on the internet.

Herxheimer reaction: Since Isolated Cleanses are oft time an aggressive approach to cleansing body organs they can release large quantities of toxins that have been within the body, especially from those that have had health problems. These released toxins can cause uncomfortable reactions as they exit the body through the bowels or skin. Some may experience digestive disruption, others rashes or other skin disorders. The general advice is to slow the cleanse by reducing or spacing the cleansing agents to find a comfortable level, but to continue the cleanse. Also consider a period of preparation with a nutritional cleanse as described above.

Other oils: Organ cleansing: Clove[C], Cumin[C], Geranium[C], Grapefruit[C], Rosemary[EC] Gastrointestinal: Lemon[C], Melaleuca[C], Oregano[C]

Detoxification Blend *(bring your body to a state of zen)*

Ingredients: Cilantro, Geranium, Juniper Berry, Rosemary, Tangerine peel

Another common formulation: Grapefruit, Helichrysum, Celery, Ledum, Hyssop and Spearmint Leaf

Addresses: Support of cleansing organs liver, kidneys, colon, lungs and skin with focus on the liver. Use with Detoxification Complex, *see* Detoxification.
(see Safety Chart, page 23)

Detoxification Blend *softgel*

Softgel: The Detoxification Blend in a handy, convenient softgel tablet for on-the-go or simple convenience.

Legend: Preferred, Suggested, Consider

Detoxification Complex

essential oils
Product A blend of whole-food extracts that supports healthy cleansing and filtering functions of the liver, kidneys, colon, lungs and skin. Use with Detoxification Blend. *See* Detoxification.

Diabetes   see also Autoimmune diseases

[Diabetic sores, Hyperglycemia, Hypoglycemia, Juvenile diabetes]

Oils: Basil[C], Coriander[C], Lavender[C] **Blends:** Grounding Blend[C], Protective Blend[C]

Diabetic conditions, as with many other serious health issues, should have treatment that includes professional medical attention.

Good eating, proper nutrition, Basic Vitality Supplements, physical activity and weight loss.

Type 2: Daily routine of 2-3 drops Grounding Blend on feet in the morning. 8-10 drops Coriander and/or Basil and 2 drops Protective Blend in capsule 1x daily. 3-5 drops Lavender on the feet at night. Consider other oils below (some are not GRAS or not for internal use). Some find it beneficial to switch oils periodically to receive all the benefits of each.

Type 1: If at onset consider the viral infection and/or the autoimmune disease protocols. Some report stabilizing/reducing insulin with Basic Vitality Supplements and detoxifying protocols. There are reports of reduction in insulin needs with very strict diets including vegan diets.

Diabetic Ulcers: 2-3 drops Lavender to area 2x daily, be consistent.

Serious Diabetic Ulcers: Use Lavender above and add Helichrysum and Frankincense at least 2x daily, be consistent. Note:This can be a very serious condition and professional medical attention should be involved.

Pre-diabetic: Basic Vitality Supplements, GI Cleansing Formula/Probiotic Defense Formula cleanse and ongoing Detoxification Blend cleanse (see Detoxification), weight management, exercise and consider Type 2 Diabetes oils if necessary.

Other oils: Cassia[C], Cinnamon Bark[C], Cypress[C], Eucalyptus[EC], Frankincense, Geranium[EC], Helichrysum, Juniper Berry[E] **Blends:** Digestive Enzyme Complex

Note: When choosing alternative oils from the list of "**Other oils:**" please review safety precautions on pages 23-28.

Diaper rash — *see also* Candidiasis

Oils: Lavender[C], Melaleuca[C] **Blends:** Grounding Blend, GI Cleansing Formula/Probiotic Defense Formula

Ointment made with 1 part each Lavender and Melaleuca with 2 parts Extra Virgin Coconut Oil. Apply after cleaning with each diaper change.

Possible root causes to consider: Candida, diet, diaper brand or fit, alcohol based and perfumed wipes.

Other oils: Frankincense, Roman Chamomile[C] **Blends:** Digestive Blend

Diarrhea

[Montezuma's revenge, Traveler's diarrhea]

Oils: Ginger[EC], Peppermint[EC] **Blends:** Digestive Blend[C]

Children/Adults: 1-5 drops Digestive Blend. Internally with capsule, water, juice, tsp of honey or agave or rub on abdomen.

Small children/sensitive skin: Dilute with carrier and rub on tummy.

Very sensitive skin: Apply to bottoms of feet.

Infants: Apply a tsp of carrier oil on the tummy followed by 1-2 drops of Digestive Blend (or one of the other listed oils). Warm hands, massage baby's tummy and lower back with circular motions. Hold and cuddle baby close afterwards. Make a warm compress with same ointment for baby after the massage and place on tummy or back. Applying ointment to feet with a foot massage is also effective.

Also consider Ginger or Peppermint to settle upset stomachs, Cinnamon Bark or Fennel for diarrhea.

Other oils: Black Pepper[EC], Cinnamon Bark[EC], Clove[E], Cumin[C], Cypress[EC], Dill[C], Fennel[C], Neroli[EC], Roman Chamomile[EC], Sandalwood[EC], Tangerine[C], Wild Orange[C]

Note: When choosing alternative oils from the list of "**Other oils:**" please review safety precautions on pages 23-28.

Diffusing

 Using a device, known as a diffuser, to disperse micro particles and the aroma of an essential oil or blend into the air. A variety of types of diffusers are available commercially.

Digestive Blend

 Ingredients: Anise, Caraway seed, Coriander, Fennel, Ginger, Peppermint, Tarragon

Another common formulation: Anise, Fennel, Ginger, Juniper, Lemongrass, Peppermint, Patchouli, Tarragon

Addresses: Congestion, constipation, diarrhea, heartburn, indigestion, motion sickness, nausea, stomachaches

(see Safety Chart, page 23)

Digestive Blend products

 Roll-on: Gentle and quick application.

Softgels: Vegetarian softgels an easy way to enjoy the benefits of the Digestive Blend.

Chewable tablets: Convenient alternative for those not able to use other application techniques.

Enzyme capsules: *see* Digestive Enzyme Complex

Cleansing assist: *see* GI Cleansing Formula

Probiotic assist: *see* Probiotic Defense Formula

Digestive conditions

Acid reflux	*see* Heartburn
Bloating	*see* Bloating
Bowel obstruction	*see* Constipation
Constipation	*see* Constipation
Diarrhea	*see* Diarrhea
Digestive cramps	*see* Stomachache
Diverticulitis	*see* Diverticulitis
Dysentery	*see* Dysentery
Flatulence	*see* Flatulence

Food poisoning	*see* Food poisoning
Gas	*see* Flatulence
Gastritis	*see* Gastroenteritis
Gastroenteritis	*see* Gastroenteritis
Indigestion	*see* Indigestion
Morning sickness	*see* Pregnancy
Motion sickness	*see* Motion sickness
Nausea	*see* Nausea
Nervous indigestion	*see* Indigestion
Stomachache (upset stomach)	*see* Stomachache
Stomach cramps	*see* Stomachache
Stomach flu	*see* Stomach flu
Ulcers	*see* Ulcers
Vomiting	*see* Vomiting

Digestive Enzyme Complex

essential oils
Product

In a vegetable capsule the Digestive Enzyme Complex is a blend of active whole food enzymes and supporting mineral cofactors that are often deficient in cooked, processed and preservative-laden foods. A Digestive Enzyme Complex includes a variety of whole food enzymes that help with digestion of proteins, fats, complex carbohydrates, sugars and fiber.

Dill *(Anethum graveolens)*

essential oil

Properties: Antibacterial, antispasmodic, antitumor, calming, digestive, disinfectant, expectorant, laxative (mild), stimulant

Addresses: ADHD, appetite modulator, bronchial mucous, colic, constipation, flatulence, head lice, headaches, hiccups, increased milk supply for nursing mothers, indigestion, liver issues, low glucose, nausea, nervousness, normalize insulin levels, pancreatic stimulant, respiratory issues

(see Safety Chart, page 23)

Legend: Preferred, Suggested, Consider

Diluting
see also Capsules, Carrier oils, Conversions, Drops

Definition Mixing an essential oil or blend with a carrier oil to reduce its strength or increase the area over which it may be applied.

Mixing chart

Carrier/ Mixture	1%	2%	5%	10%
1 teaspoon	1 drop	2 drops	5 drops	10 drops
1 Tablespoon	3 drops	6 drops	15 drops	30 drops
1 fluid oz	6 drops	12 drops	30 drops	60 drops

Disc degeneration
see Back conditions

Disinfectants
see also Household care

Disinfectants are antimicrobial substances that are applied to non-living areas to destroy microorganisms. A partial list below:

Blends: Cleansing Blend[C], Protective Blend[C]

Oils: Arborvitae[C], Birch[C], Douglas Fir[C], Eucalyptus[EC], Grapefruit[C], Green Mandarin[C], Invigorating Blend[C], Lavender[EC], Lemon[C], Litsea[C], Melaleuca[C]

Diuretic

This is a partial list of oils and blends with diuretic properties:

Black Pepper[E], Cedarwood[EC], Copaiba[C], Cypress[EC], Dougla Fir[C], Fennel[EC], Grapefruit[C], Green Mandarin[C], Juniper Berry[EC], Lavender[EC], Lemon[C], Lemongrass[C], Rosemary[EC], Wild Orange, Invigorating Blend[C]

Diverticulitis

Oils: Ginger[C], Peppermint **Blends:** Digestive Blend[C], GI Cleansing Formula/Probiotic Defense Formula

2-4 drops Digestive Blend, Ginger or Peppermint 2x daily in a capsule.

Long term: Periodic cleanse with GI Cleansing Formula/Probiotic Defense Formula and Detoxification Blend products, Fiber in diet, Basic Vitality Supplements.

Other oils: Cinnamon Bark[C], Clove[C], Lavender[C] **Blends/Products:** Detoxification Blend and Detoxification Complex

Dizziness   *see* Vertigo

Dog care

Oils: Frankincense **Blends:** Digestive Blend, Protective Blend, Respiratory Blend, Restful Blend

The following reported results:
  Anxiety: Restful Blend or Grounding Blend with Lavender
  Cuts and Wounds: Lavender, Melaleuca (dilute), Protective Blend
  Digestive problems: Digestive Blend or Peppermint
  Fungal infection: Protective Blend
  Respiratory: Respiratory Blend
  Seizures: Frankincense
  Tumor/growth: Frankincense
  Warts: Protective Blend

Common application technique: Few drops diluted on paws or topically to area for cuts, infections, tumors. Some report Melaleuca should be highly diluted.

Oils to avoid: Birch, Camphor, Oregano and Wintergreen.
Other oils: Lavender, Melaleuca, Peppermint **Blends:** Grounding Blend

Douglas Fir *(Pseudotsuga menziesii)*

essential oil

Properties: Analgesic, antioxidant, antiseptic, astringent, diuretic, expectorant

Addresses: Arthritic pain, asthma, bronchitis, cold and flu, congestion, cuts and wounds, joint pain, muscle pain, stress

(see Safety Chart, page 23)

Drops   *see also* Capsules, Conversions

Definition

A drop is a common measure used when applying and mixing essential oils. A drop is basically the amount of oil that comes out of an essential oils bottle with a reducer insert in the top that restricts the flow and allows the oils to come out slowly a

Legend: Preferred, Suggested, Consider

drop at a time. It is not a precise measurement since drop size varies from oil to oil depending on a number of factors. An average number of drops per milliliter is 20. The chart below shows how this varies with some common oils.

Essential Oil	Drops in 5 ml (ave)
Lemon	85
Melaleuca	87
Oregano	120
Frankincense	124
Sandalwood	135
Peppermint	140

Drugs   *see* Addictions

Dry cough   *see* Cough

Dry lips   *see* Chapped lips

Dry skin   *see* Chapped skin

Duodenal ulcer   *see* Ulcers

Dust mites   *see* Allergies, Insect repellent, Scabies

DVT (deep vein thrombosis)   *see* Blood clots

Dysentery   *see also* Amoebic Dysentery

Oils: Cinnamon Bark, Lavender[C], Lemon, Oregano **Blends:** Digestive Blend, Protective Blend

Mild: 2-3 drops Lavender in capsule 2x daily

Moderate: 3-5 drops each Digestive Blend and Protective Blend (or Cinnamon Bark, Oregano) to a capsule and take 3x per day. 2-4 weeks may be required.

More difficult: Use same capsule protocol above but a rectal application 2x daily.

Prevention during travel: 2 drops each Lemon and Protective Blend in mouthful of water 1-2x daily.

Other oils: Melaleuca, Roman Chamomile, Thyme

Note: Dysentery can come from Bacterial, Viral or Parasitic infection. If you know the type then moderate the above suggestions to use oils known to be effective against that type of infection. See Antibacterial, Antiparasitic, Antiviral.

Dyslexia

Oils: Frankincense, Lemon, Peppermint

1-2 drop each Frankincense, Lemon, Peppermint internally in capsule. Some suggest using oils under tongue or topically on brain stem or suboccipital triangle. Experiment with drops, application and frequency. Use Basic Vitality Supplements consistently.

Other oils: Vetiver[C] **Blends/Products:** Basic Vitality Supplements, Focus Blend[C]

Dysmenorrhoea *(cramps or painful menstrual periods)*
see also Hormonal balance

Oils: Clary Sage[EC], Cypress[EC], Peppermint[EC], Rosemary[EC] **Blends/Products:** Monthly Blend for Women, Phytoestrogen Complex, Tension Blend

Phytoestrogen Complex and Monthly Blend for Women are specifically formulated to support hormone balance and manage menstrual discomfort. 1-3 drops of Monthly Blend for Women or Tension Blend topically to abdomen.

Also suggested are 2-4 drops each Cypress and Rosemary topically to abdomen. Warm compress on abdomen after applying oils. Also consider Basil, Clary Sage, Geranium or Peppermint applied topically to lower abdomen or lower back. For additional help cup & inhale and use warm compress after applying oils. (Note: Noted experts and many others point out that different oils work for different folks and there is usually a need to do some experimentation to determine what works best for each individual).

Other oils: Basil[C], Geranium[C], Jasmine[EC], Sandalwood

Dyspepsia	*see* Indigestion

Dysphagia	*see* Swallowing difficulty

Notes:

Legend: Preferred, Suggested, Consider

E. coli enteritis   *see* Food poisoning

Ear conditions

Earache   *see* Earache
Hearing loss   *see* Hearing loss
Meniere's disease   *see* Meniere's disease
Tinnitus   *see* Tinnitus

Earache

Oils: Basil[EC], Grapefruit[C], Lavender[EC]

3 drops Basil on 1/2 of one side of cotton ball, push lightly into ear with oil side to outside. You may also want to place warm wash cloth over ear. Add more Basil to the cotton ball every 2-3 hours.

Oregano is too "hot" to use with a cotton ball or around ear but it or other oils may be applied on bottoms of feet. 1-3 drops every 2-3 hours.

Added pain relief: Rub few drops Grapefruit behind and around outer part of the ear. With ear infection there is a good possibility lymph nodes are inflamed. Lightly massage with Frankincense, Grapefruit with a carrier oil from under ear, down length of neck towards heart.

Other oils: Frankincense[C], Lemon[EC], Lime[C], Melaleuca[C], Oregano, **Blends:** Cleansing Blend[C]

Eating conditions

Addictions   *see* Addictions
Anorexia   *see* Anorexia
Appetite, loss of   *see* Anorexia
Bulimia   *see* Bulimia
Overeating   *see* Weight loss
Weight loss   *see* Weight loss

Ecthyma
see also Impetigo

Oils: Frankincense, Helichrysum, Oregano **Blends:** GI Cleansing Formula

Clean area with Protective Blend Foaming Wash. 2 drops each of Frankincense and Oregano topically to area. Dilute with carrier oil to reduce stinging if necessary. If a child is apprehensive let them inhale Lavender to relax them. Allow oils to absorb then cover. Repeat 3x daily. Cleanse hands with Protective Blend Foaming Wash to prevent spreading infection.

1-3 GI Cleansing Formula capsules or 3-5 drops Oregano in capsule 1x daily depending on age. Continue until scabs clear and new skin appears; then continue 1-2 weeks with 2 drops each Frankincense and Helichrysum applied topically to promote the healing and reduce scarring.

Other oils: Lavender[C] **Blends:** Protective Blend Foaming Hand Wash

Eczema (dermatitis)
see also Psoriasis

Oils: Frankincense[C], Geranium[EC], Helichrysum[C], Lavender[EC], Melaleuca[C], Roman Chamomile[EC] **Blends:** GI Cleansing Formula/Probiotic Defense Formula, Topical Blend[C]

Topical Blend or self-made blend using 10 drops Lavender, 5 drops each Helichrysum and Myrrh, 3-5 drops Melaleuca with 1 tsp EVCO. Apply topically to area.

Emotional: Also consider Lavender or Jasmine has been mentioned.

Candida or other internal: Also cleanses may be necessary. GI Cleansing Formula/Probiotic Defense Formula, Detoxification Blend or 2-3 drops Lemon with each glass of water.

Other oils: Bergamot[EC], Birch[C], Copaiba[C], Jasmine[C], Juniper Berry[EC], Myrrh, Yarrow[C] **Blends/Products:** Basic Vitality Supplements

Edema (swelling, water retention)

Oils: Cypress[C], Grapefruit[C], Lemon[C], Lemongrass[C] **Blends:** Basic Vitality Supplements

Massage 2-4 drops Cypress or Lemongrass with 4-6 drops of Lemon or Grapefruit directly to area of swelling with a grape seed or other carrier oil. Massage with motions towards the heart. Repeat 2-3 times daily. Couple with Basic Vitality Supplements and 1-3 drops Lemon to glass of water 4x daily.

Other oils: Cedarwood[C], Geranium[EC], Patchouli[E], Rosemary[C], Tangerine[C]
Blends: Invigorating Blend[C]

Elemi *(Canarium luzonicum)*

Properties: Antibacterial, antidepressant, antifungal, anti-infectious, antiseptic, antiviral, decongestant, expectorant, sedative

Addresses: Bronchitis, chapped skin, Congestion, coughs, cuts, emotional fatigue, mature skin, rashes, sinus infection, stress, wrinkles

(see Safety Chart, page 23)

Emergency preparedness   *see also* Water purification

Suggested oils and blends for an Emergency Preparedness Kit:

5 oil kit: Lavender, Lemon, Peppermint; Protective Blend, Respiratory Blend

10 oil kit: Digestive Blend, Frankincense, Lavender, Lemon, Melaleuca, Oregano, Peppermint; Protective Blend, Respiratory Blend, Soothing Blend

15 oil kit: Cleansing Blend, Clove, Digestive Blend, Frankincense, Lavender, Lemon, Lemongrass, Massage Blend, Melaleuca, Oregano, Peppermint; Protective Blend, Repellent Blend, Respiratory Blend, Soothing Blend

Emotional conditions   *see also* Mental conditions or Personality disorders

Agitation	*see* Irritability
Anxiety (fear)	*see* Anxiety
Apathy	*see* Mood swings
Bipolar (manic depressive)	*see* Bipolar
Calming	*see* Anxiety
Depression (despair)	*see* Depression
Fatigue	*see* Depression

Grief (sorrow)	*see* Emotional strength
Hysteria	*see* Mood swings
Irritability (anger)	*see* Irritability
Mood swings	*see* Mood swings
Nervousness	*see* Anxiety
OCD	*see* OCD
Panic attack	*see* Anxiety
Paranoia	*see* Paranoia
PTSD	*see* Stress
Restlessness	*see* Anxiety
Sadness	*see* Anxiety
Strength	*see* Emotional strength
Stress (tension)	*see* Stress
Suicide	*see* Depression

Emotional strength

Oils: Frankincense, Geranium, Neroli, Ylang Ylang **Blends:** Cleansing Blend, Comforting Blend, Encouraging Blend, Grounding Blend, Inspiring Blend, Invigorating Blend, Joyful Blend, Reassuring Blend, Renewing Blend, Restful Blend, Uplifting Blend

Suggestions made by others include using oils or blends in a roller bottle and apply behind ears, on wrists, bottoms of the feet and/or along spine 2-3x daily. Others diffuse or use cup & inhale.

Acceptance: Grounding Blend, Joyful Blend, Renewing Blend

Anger: Grapefruit, Neroli, Patchouli, Grounding Blend, Renewing Blend, Restful Blend, *see also* Irritability

Change, dealing with: Comforting Blend, Invigorating Blend, Restful Blend

Courage: Encouraging Blend, Grounding Blend

Emotional foundation: Inspiring Blend, Invigorating Blend, Joyful Blend, Restful Blend

Emotional protection: Frankincense

Emotional release: Geranium highly recommended plus Basil, Cassia, Cypress, Melissa, Neroli, Protective Blend, Renewing Blend

Feminine energy: Encouraging Blend, Ylang Ylang or Sandalwood

Forgiveness: Grounding Blend, Renewing Blend, Restful Blend

Grief: Geranium, Grounding Blend, Joyful Blend, Reassuring Blend, Restful Blend, Uplifting Blend

Honesty: Cleansing Blend

Joy: Joyful Blend or Invigorating Blend

Motivation: Encouraging Blend, Joyful Blend

Nurturing: Ylang Ylang, Reassuring Blend, Restful Blend

Passion: Inspiring Blend, Invigorating Blend, Joyful Blend

Reinitialize: Grounding Blend, Invigorating Blend

Responsibility: Grounding Blend, Massage Blend, Grounding Blend/ Vetiver

Self Confidence: Frankincense, Frankincense/Peppermint, Grounding Blend, Grounding Blend/Vetiver, Inspiring Blend

Self Image: Inspiring Blend, Restful Blend

Self Love: Grounding Blend, Restful Blend

Other oils: Basil, Cassia, Cumin[C], Cypress, Melissa, Sandalwood, Tangerine[C], Vetiver **Blends:** Massage Blend, Protective Blend

Emotions, helping negative

Some have suggested using one or more of 6 basic emotional blends for help with negative feelings as suggested below:

Discouraged: Encouraging Blend

Gloomy: Encouraging Blend and/or Uplifing Blend

Distressed: Uplifing Blend

Somber: Uplifting Blend

Disinterested: Uplifing Blend and/or Inspring Blend

Bored: Inspring Blend

Discontented: Inspiring Blend

Bitter: Inspiring Blend and/or Renewing Blend

Angry: Renewing Blend

Ashamed: Renewing Blend

Sad: Renewing Blend and/or Comforting Blend

Grieving: Comforting Blend

Hurt: Comforting Blend

Worried: Comforting Blend and/or Reassuring Blend

Fearful: Reassuring Blend

Anxious: Reassuring Blend

Insecure: Reassuring Blend and/or Encouraging Blend

Apathetic: Encouraging Blend

Diffuse, cup & inhale or topically to back of neck, wrists or over heart.

Emphysema

Oils: Eucalyptus[EC], Frankincense[C], Lemon **Blends:** Respiratory Blend

To help open airways 3-5 drops Respiratory Blend (or Eucalyptus with carrier) topically to chest and diffused or near nostrils on upper lip or on hands to cup over nostrils at sleep time. 1-2 drops Grounding Blend on feet as well. During day drink water with 1-2 drops Lemon or Wild Orange per glass. Basic Vitality Supplements will also help.

Other oils: Blue Tansy[E], Cinnamon Bark[E], Cypress[C], Peppermint, Thyme[E]
Blends/ Products: Basic Vitality Supplements, Grounding Blend[C]

Encouraging Blend

essential oils **Blend** (comes in a roll-on dispenser)

Ingredients: Basil, Clementine, Coriander, Melissa, Peppermint, Rosemary, Vanilla, Yuzu

Addresses: An emotional health blend to motivate and encourage.

(see Safety Chart, page 23)

Endometriosis   *see also* Hormonal balance

Oils: Clary Sage[C], Frankincense[C], Sandalwood **Blends/Products:** Monthly Blend for Women, Phytoestrogen Complex

Phytoestrogen Complex and Monthly Blend for Women are specifically formulated to balance hormones and manage menstrual problems. Place 2-3 drops Frankincense under tongue every night and every morning. For pain and cramps 8-12 drops Sandalwood in capsule at outset, second day taper to 6-8 drops Sandalwood in capsule.

Other oils: Cypress[C], Geranium[C], Rosemary **Blends:** Protective Blend[C]

Legend: Preferred, Suggested, Consider

Energy & Stamina Complex   *see also* Supplements

essential oils
Product

An Energy & Stamina Complex supports healthy mitochondrial function and aerobic capacity and improves stamina naturally without the use of harmful stimulants. Use Energy & Stamina Complex as a healthy long-term alternative to caffeinated drinks and supplements for increased energy and vitality.

Energy, lack of   *see* Fatigue, physical

Enlarged prostate (prostatitis)   *see* Prostate conditions

Enlightening Blend (a Yoga blend)

essential oils
Blend

Ingredients: Lemon Peel, Grapefruit Peel, Siberian Fir, Osmanthus Flower, Melissa Leaf

Addresses: Promotes feelings of happiness, clarity and courage and encourages rising to achieve goals and improved performance.

(see Safety Chart, page 23)

Epilepsy

Oils: Bergamot[C], Frankincense[C] **Blends:** Grounding Blend, Restful Blend

2-3 drops Frankincense and Bergamot morning and evening to bottoms of feet and at brain stem. For calming and balance: Grounding Blend in morning, Restful Blend in evening. It is beneficial to rotate with other oils of similar properties periodically to get the additional benefits of each.

Weekly do the Massage Blend Technique (replace Protective Blend with Cinnamon Bark/Clove/Wild Orange blend and Soothing Blend with Helichrysum/Peppermint blend), Basic Vitality Supplements.

Precaution: Epilepsy, as with many other health issues, should have treatment that includes professional medical attention. Oils to avoid Basil, Birch, Dill, Fennel, Rosemary and Wintergreen or blends containing these oils. [Also mentioned from other sources are these oils to avoid or to use with care: Camphor, Eucalyptus, Fennel, Galbanum, Hyssop, Nutmeg, Pennyroyal, Sage, Savin, Spike Lavender (not the common Lavender angustifolia), Tansy (not to be confused with Blue Tansy), Tarragon,

Thuja, Thujone, Turpentine, Wormwood.]

Note: Soothing Blend has Camphor and Wintergreen and Protective Blend has Eucalyptus and Rosemary.

Other oils: Clary Sage[C], Clove[C], Thyme[EC] **Blends/Products:** Basic Vitality Supplements, Massage Blend

Epstein-Barr
see also Mononucleosis

Oils: Frankincense, Lemon, Thyme[E] **Blends:** Grounding Blend, Protective Blend[C]

Symptoms: Grounding Blend (or other calming oils) diffused or inhaled directly.

Viral infection: 3 drops each Frankincense, Lemon, Protective Blend, Thyme in capsule 3x daily.

Other oils: Lavender, Oregano[E] **Blends:** Joyful Blend, Restful Blend

Equilibrium
see Vertigo

Erectile dysfunction
see also Aphrodisiac, Libido

Oils: Basil, Clary Sage[EC], Coriander, Cypress, Geranium, Sandalwood[EC], Ylang Ylang **Blends/Products:** Basic Vitality Supplements

Following is a summary of what others have suggested:

Nutritional balance: Basic Vitality Supplements used consistently.

Hormonal balance/sexual stimulants: Anti-Aging Blend applied topically to genital area or Clary Sage, Sandalwood, Ylang Ylang applied topically, inhaled or taken internally.

Circulation improvement: Coriander, Cypress. Apply topically with dilution.

Anxiety/Stress: Basil, Lavender, Ylang Ylang. Inhale using cup & inhale, diffusion or few drops on pillow.

Other oils: Black Pepper, Frankincense, Lavender **Blends:** Anti-Aging Blend

Esophagitis
see Swallowing difficulty

Legend: Preferred, Suggested, Consider

Essential Ointment

Product

An ointment including essential oils know to help in soothing skin irritations: Cedarwood, Frankincense, Helichrysum, Lavender and Melaleuca. Added to this are ingredients to provide a moisture barrier and hydration of the skin to assure protection as the skin returns to a healthy state.

Essential tremors

Oils: Frankincense, Rosemary **Blends:** Basic Vitality Supplements, Grounding Blend

1-2 drops Frankincense under tongue and 1-2 drops along spine daily. Cypress and/or Rosemary are reported to help. Use Basic Vitality Supplements consistently and avoid artificial sweeteners.

Anxiety/Stress: Diffuse or hand massage Grounding Blend or Lavender.

Other oils: Cypress, Helichrysum, Lavender, Peppermint **Blends:** Massage Blend

Esters   see Chemical constituents

Estrogen   see Hormonal balance

Eucalyptus (Eucalyptus radiata)

essential oil

Properties: Analgesic, antibacterial, antibiotic, anti-inflammatory, antiseptic, antiviral, disinfectant, expectorant

Addresses: Arthritic pain, asthma, back pain, bronchitis, burns, cold and flu, congestion, cough, cuts and wounds, diarrhea, earache, fever, herpes, indigestion, migraines, stomachache

(see Safety Chart, page 23)

EVCO *Extra Virgin Coconut Oil*   *see also* **FCO**

 Def**inition**   The terms Extra Virgin Coconut Oil and Virgin Coconut Oil are used interchangeably to refer to coconut oil that has been cold-pressed soon after the coconut is harvested. In the liquid state the oil is clear and smells and tastes like coconut. Some commercial grade coconut oil is bleached to be clear but lacks the smell and taste of coconut.

Exfoliating   *see* Personal care and Skin care

Exhaustion   *see* Fatigue

Expectorant   *see* Cough

Eye conditions

Cataracts	*see* Eyesight failing
Conjunctivitis (pink eye)	*see* Conjunctivitis
Corneal ulcer	*see* Eyesight failing
Eyesight, failing (presbyopia)	*see* Eyesight failing
Glaucoma	*see* Eyesight failing
Inflammation	*see* Eye injury or discomfort
Itchy	*see* Eye injury or discomfort
Macular degeneration	*see* Eyesight failing
Redness	*see* Eye injury or discomfort
Retinal detachment	*see* Eyesight failing
Sty	*see* Sty
Uveitis (iritis)	*see* Eyesight failing
Vision, improve	*see* Eyesight failing

Eye injury or discomfort   *see also* Conjunctivitis

[Inflammation, Itchy, Redness]

Essential oils must not be used directly in the eye. They will not injure the eye but there will be very uncomfortable stinging. If this happens do not flush the eye with water, rather use FCO or olive oil.

For redness caused by allergies use the oils and techniques suggested under allergies. If an eye infection, bruise or trauma, use oils commonly suggested for such problems but apply them as suggested in the following:

Older children/adults: 2-3 drops around socket of eye by putting oils in hand, apply with finger tip.

Younger children: Use hard shell eye patch (pharmacy) with 2 drops of oils on 1/3 of a cotton pad placed in patch with oils side of cotton away from eye. Place over affected eye. Also apply oils on reflexology points.

Caution children not to rub eyes and with small children when oils are put on feet, place socks on feet so oils are not accidentally transferred to eyes.

Eyesight, failing

[Cataracts, Corneal ulcer, Eyesight failing (Presbyopia), Glaucoma, Macular degeneration, Retinal detachment, Uveitis (Iriitis)]

Oils: Cypress, Frankincense[C], Helichrysum, Lavender[C] **Blends:** Anti-Aging Blend[C]

Helping and regeneration: 1-2 drops Anti-Aging Blend, Helichrysum or Frankincense in roller bottle or on end of finger and dab around eye socket (not in eye) 2-3x daily. Additionally, or in case of sensitivity, rub oils on reflexology point for eyes 2-3x daily.

Infection (uveitis or inflammation): Use Anti-Aging Blend or equal parts Frankincense, Cypress and Lavender (in roller bottle), apply around eye socket as above but increase frequency to 3-4x daily and continue for a few days after infection clears.

Other oils: Rosemary[EC], Sandalwood[C], Ylang Ylang

Notes:

Legend: Preferred, Suggested, Consider

F

Facial fine lines
see Wrinkles

Facial neuralgia
see Neuralgia

Failed back syndrome
see Back conditions

Failing eyesight
see Eyesight, failing

Fainting

Oils: Peppermint[E], Rosemary[EC]

With person in prone position and feet raised higher than heart, loosen tight clothing. Have them inhale Rosemary or Peppermint to gain clarity and focus more quickly. 2-3 drops on a tissue or your hand and let them inhale or directly from bottle if they are able. Encourage them to get up slowly when ready.

If they do not respond in a short time, consider it a medical emergency and take proper action.

If the fainting is due to a known condition, refer to the underlying condition to help with essential oils.

Other oils: Basil[EC], Black Pepper[E], Lavender[EC]

Fatigue, emotional
see Depression
see also Chronic Fatigue Syndrome

Fatigue, mental
see Mental acuity
see also Chronic Fatigue Syndrome

Fatigue, physical *(exhaustion, weakness)*
see also Chronic Fatigue Syndrome

Oils: Peppermint[EC], Rosemary[EC] **Blends/Products:** Basic Vitality Supplements, Joyful Blend[C], Massage Blend

4-6 drops Peppermint into hand, pull palm across back of neck and

---

Safety charts ... page 23   Special cautions ... page 3   129

massage, then pull palm half-way up the back of head. Repeating hourly or more often if desired.

Or put Joyful Blend, Peppermint or blend of Peppermint and Rosemary in an inhaler, inhale as necessary if experiencing drowsiness.

To help restore balance in all body functions, use Basic Vitality Supplements consistently and the Massage Blend Technique periodically.

Other oils: Basil[EC], Cinnamon Bark[EC], Eucalyptus[EC], Frankincense[EC], Lavender[EC], Lemon[EC], Petitgrain[C], Pink Pepper[C], Spikenard[C]

FCO *Fractionated Coconut Oil* — *see also* **EVCO**

Definition Smaller fatty acids and long-chain triglycerides are separated from the whole coconut oil leaving only saturated fats. This is known as Fractionated Coconut Oil. This oil never goes rancid, is clear, is odorless, absorbs well into the skin, no greasy feel, mixes well with other oils, does not irritate or aggravate problem skin and is fully digestible. These properties make FCO an ideal carrier oil to mix with essential oils and blends.

Fear — *see* Anxiety

Female related conditions

Hormonal balance	*see* Hormonal balance
Hot flashes	*see* Hot flashes
Menopause	*see* Menopause
Menstruation	*see* Menstrual conditions
PMS (premenstrual syndrome)	*see* PMS
Premenopause	*see* Premenopause

Fennel (Foeniculum vulgare)

essential oil

Properties: Anti-inflammatory, antioxidant, antiparasitic, antiseptic, antispasmodic, astringent, digestive, diuretic, expectorant

Addresses: Constipation, diarrhea, flatulence, hormonal balance, indigestion, kidney failure, lactation, menstrual problems, nausea, PMS, skin care, stomachache, weight loss

(see Safety Chart, page 23)

Legend: Preferred, Suggested, Consider

Fertility   *see* Infertility

Fever

Oils: Eucalyptus[EC], Lemon[EC], Peppermint[EC]

1-2 drops Peppermint to forehead, back of neck and bottoms of feet. Apply frequently, 15-30 minutes, until fever goes down. Also tepid compress or bath with Peppermint or Eucalyptus.

Infants: 1 drop diluted 3:1 on forehead and back of neck. Be careful baby does not touch areas and rub eyes. Or 1 drop Peppermint on caregiver's hands, let evaporate until moisture disappears, rub on baby's feet.

Other oils: Arborvitae[C], Basil[EC], Black Pepper[C], Frankincense[EC], Lavender[C], Lime[C], Siberian Fir[C], Yarrow[C]

Fever blister   *see* Cold sores

Fibrillation   *see* Heart conditions

Fibromyalgia   *see also* Autoimmune diseases

Oils: Helichrysum[C], Lavender[C] **Blends/Products:** Basic Vitality Supplements, Detoxification Blend/Detoxification Complex, GI Cleansing Formula/Probiotic Defense Formula, Grounding Blend, Massage Blend, Restful Blend, Soothing Blend[C]

Experiences from others include addressing at multiple levels:

Pain: Soothing Blend or Massage Blend topically to points of discomfort. Frequent use of the Massage Blend Technique.

Detoxification: Detoxification Blend/Detoxification Complex and/or GI Cleansing Formula/Probiotic Defense Formula. *See* Detoxification

Strengthen Immune System: Apply the Massage Blend Technique frequently.

Nutritional balance: Basic Vitality Supplements and eliminate harmful foods and habits.

Emotional support: Restful Blend, Grounding Blend. S*ee also*

Emotional conditions

Other oils: Copaiba^C, Melaleuca^C, Oregano^C, Thyme^EC

| **Fingernail fungus** | *see* Nail fungus |

| **Fingernails, strengthen** | *see* Nails, strengthen |

| **Fir, Douglas** | *see* Douglas Fir |

| **Fir, Siberian** | *see* Siberian Fir |

| **Fish poisoning** | *see* Food poisoning |

Flabby skin

Oils: Cypress^C, Grapefruit^C, Lavender^C **Blends:** Metabolic Blend

Cellulite: Topically apply Grapefruit then layer with Metabolic Blend to locations.

Tone/Condition: Skin Care products Anti-Aging Moisturizer, Tightening Serum and Invigorating Scrub (*see* Skin care). Self-made blend of 18-36 drops Lavender with 1 oz EVCO and 1/2 oz wheat germ oil.

Other oils: Frankincense, Geranium, Helichrysum

| **Flat warts** | *see* Warts |

Flatulence (gas)

Oils: Black Pepper^EC, Ginger^EC, Lavender^EC, Peppermint^EC, Roman Chamomile^EC **Blends:** Digestive Blend^C

1-3 drops Digestive Blend or Ginger in capsule 15-30 minutes before meal. Also apply oils to abdomen or reflexology points on feet. Each person and food is different; experiment with different oils.

For chronic problems consider the GastroIntestinal Tract cleanse detailed under Detoxification.

Other oils: Bergamot^EC, Cardamom^EC, Cilantro^C, Coriander^EC, Cumin^C, Dill^C, Fennel^E, Marjoram^E, Rosemary^EC, Spikenard^C, Yarrow^C **Blends/**

Products: Detoxification Blend, Detoxification Complex, Digestive Enzyme Complex[C], GI Cleansing Formula, Probiotic Defense Formula

Fleas

Oils: Lavender **Blends:** Cleansing Blend, Repellent Blend[C]

Dab Lavender (Cleansing Blend or Repellent Blend) topically directly on areas bitten as soon as possible. Repeat every 1-2 hours until symptoms disappear. For young children or very sensitive skin dilute oils with a carrier, probably not necessary with Lavender. Avoid scratching as much as possible.

Other oils: Lemongrass, Peppermint

Flu (Influenza)   see also Stomach flu

[Bird flu, H1N1/swine flu, West Nile, H3N2]

Oils: Frankincense[C], Lemon[EC], Oregano[C] **Blends:** Protective Blend[C], Protective Blend+ Softgels[C], Protective Blend Foaming Hand Wash

Virus: Protective Blend+ capsules 2x daily or 5 drops Protective Blend, 8 drops Oregano and 3 drops Frankincense in capsule (quantities for adults w/o sensitivities) 2x daily. Begin oils as soon as symptoms are detected. Then taper down quantities as symptoms subside and continue until all lingering symptoms are gone.

1 drop Oregano, 2 drops Protective Blend, and 2 drops Lemon in Tbsp water, gargle 1-2 minutes 2x daily and swallow. (Oregano is "hot".)

Children: If unable to take internally open Protective Blend+ capsule and dilute or dilute above blend and rub on feet and chest.

Prevent spreading: Diffuse Protective Blend, clean common use areas with Protective Blend Hand Wash.

Other oils: Eucalyptus[EC], Lavender[EC], Melaleuca[C], Peppermint[EC], Ravensara[C], Rosemary[EC], Star Anise[C], Thyme[EC] **Blends:** Respiratory Blend[C]

Note: When choosing alternative oils from the list of "**Other oils:**" please review safety precautions on pages 23-28.

Focus   see Mental acuity

Focus Blend *(become in tune with yourself)*

essential oils
Blend

(comes in roll-on)

Ingredients: Amyris bark, Frankincense, Lime, Patchouli, Roman Chamomile, Sandalwood (Hawaiian), Ylang Ylang

Addresses: Restore focus, stay on task, clarity, alertness, clear thoughts

(see Safety Chart, page 23)

Focus Blend for Children   *see* Kid's Blends

Food allergies   *see also* Allergies and Food intolerance

[Eggs, Fish, Lactose, Nuts, Other foods]

Oils: Lavender, Lemon, Melaleuca, Peppermint **Blends:** Digestive Blend

To relieve symptoms: Lemon/Lavender/Peppermint for nasal itching (see Allergies), Lavender and Melaleuca topically for eczema and skin problems, Digestive Blend for digestive discomfort.

Some suggest an elimination diet to determine what foods to avoid. Basic Vitality Supplements are important in maintaining proper nutrition.

Other Blends/Products: Basic Vitality Supplements

Food intolerance   *see also* Allergies, Food allergies and Celiac disease (Gluten intolerance)

[Lactose and other foods intolerance]

Blends/Products: Digestive Blend, Digestive Enzyme Complex, GI Cleansing Formula, Probiotic Defense Formula

Use a GI Cleansing Formula/Probiotic Defense Formula cleanse and Digestive Enzyme Complex capsule with each meal or as needed. For symptom relief use Digestive Blend topically on tummy area.

Some suggest an elimination diet to determine what foods to avoid. Basic Vitality Supplements are important in maintaining proper nutrition.

Other oils: Lemon, Lavender, Peppermint **Blends/Products:** Basic Vitality Supplements

Food poisoning   *see also* Diarrhea, Dysentery, Stomach flu

[Botulism, Campylobacter enteritis, Cholera, E. coli enteritis, Fish poisoning, Giardia, Listeria, Salmonella, Shigella, Staphylococcus aureus]

Oils: Ginger, Oregano, Peppermint **Blends:** Digestive Blend[C], Protective Blend[C]

Symptoms/infection: 3-4 drops Digestive Blend internally in capsule 3x daily. May also be applied topically to lower stomach area.

Babies/children: Apply topically with carrier oil.

Infants: Apply to bottoms of feet with carrier oil.

Additional help: 5 drops Protective Blend, 3 drops Cinnamon Bark, Oregano or Thyme 3x per day in capsule for infection. Ginger and Peppermint to settle upset stomachs. Cinnamon Bark or Cassia topically to lower stomach with carrier for diarrhea.

Other oils: Cassia, Cinnamon Bark, Fennel, Sandalwood, Thyme

Foot odor
see Body odor

Forgetfulness
see Memory

Forgiveness
see Emotional strength

Fortifying Blend

(comes in roll-on)

Blend

Ingredients: Buddha Wood, Balsam Fir Wood, Black Pepper Fruit, Hinoki, and Patchouli essential oils with Cocoa Extract in a base of Fractionated Coconut Oil

Addresses: Anxiety, emotional strength and stability, uplift mood, skin blemishes, skin care

(see Safety Chart, page 23)

Fractionated coconut oil
see FCO

Fracture
see Bone, broken

Frankincense *(Boswellia frereana)*

essential oil (also available in a roll-on)

Properties: Analgesic, antidepressant, antifungal, anti-inflammatory, antiseptic, astringent, diuretic, expectorant, sedative

Addresses: Asthma, bronchitis, cold and flu, cuts and wounds, dermatitis, immune strengthener, indigestion, neurological disorders, scarring, skin disorders, sore throat, stress, stomachache, tumor reduction

Free radicals
see Antioxidant

Frigidity
see Aphrodisiac or Libido

Frostbite
see also Chilblains

Oils: Helichrysum, Peppermint **Blends:** Massage Blend

1-2 drops Massage Blend to affected area, massage lightly. Follow with 1-2 drops Helichrysum, apply warm compress. Repeat 2x daily. If Massage Blend not available use Cypress, Lavender and Marjoram.

2 -3 drops Peppermint every 3-4 hours to stimulate circulation.

Other oils: Cypress[C], Lavender[C], Marjoram

Fruit and vegetable cleaning
see Household care

Fruit and Veggie Drink Mix

Product

This mix is a blend of fruits and vegetables known to be high in vitamins, minerals and nutrients that are helpful supplements to modern diets. Available in a powdered form to easily complement meals and provide supplement nutrition.

Fungal infections
see also Antifungal

Athlete's foot	*see* Athlete's foot
Candida	*see* Candida
Jock itch	*see* Jock itch
Nail fungus	*see* Nail fungus
Ringworm	*see* Ringworm
Valley fever	*see* Valley fever

Legend: Preferred, Suggested, Consider

Gallbladder inflammation (cholecystitis)   see also Gallstones

Oils: Lemon, Peppermint **Blends/Products:** Detoxification Blend, Detoxification Complex, Digestive Blend, Protective Blend, Probiotic Defense Formula

Discomfort and pain (also to help those with gallbladder removed with digestive discomfort):

2-4 drops each Digestive Blend and Peppermint topically to abdomen or internally in capsule. Alternate between oils. Also regular Probiotic Defense Formula.

Long term detoxification and balance:

The "heavy duty" cleanse below has been suggested. Avoid or reduce quantities of oils if uncomfortable reactions are encountered.

Do 14 day cleanse using: 10 drops Peppermint, 10 drops Lemon, 2 drops Protective Blend, juice of 1 lemon. Add to 8 oz water, drink over one hour period.

Follow with daily Detoxification Blend detoxification: 2 tablets Detoxification Complex morning and evening, 5 drops Detoxification Blend internally in capsule daily.

Other oils: Geranium[C], Helichrysum[C], Lavender[C], Rose[E], Rosemary[EC], Yarrow[C]

Gallstones   see also Gallbladder inflammation

Oils: Lemon[E], Rosemary[EC] **Blends:** Detoxification Blend[C], Digestive Blend

Some report success with Detoxification Blend, other protocols follow:

To eliminate gallstones:

Prepare the following mixture: 1/2 cup high quality olive oil, 2-6 drops Lemon, 1/2 squeezed lemon; warm before adding essential oil.

Drink mixture with straw before retiring to bed. On retiring, curl up on right side.

For pain relief:
1 Tbsp castor oil with 3-5 drops Digestive Blend applied over gallbladder area and cover with dry cloth and heating pad.

Or 2 drops Lavender to water bottle, shake and sip.

To help prevent gallstones (from forming if you are prone):
1-2 drops Lemon to each glass of water during day (6-8).

Other oils: Geranium[C], Grapefruit[C], Lavender[E], Lime[C]

Ganglion cyst
see also Cysts

Oils: Oregano, Thyme

2 drops Oregano topically on cyst in mornings (dilute if necessary), 2 drops Thyme topically on cyst in evening. Repeat daily until gone.

Other oils: Frankincense[C]

Gas
see Flatulence

Gastric ulcer
see Ulcers

Gastritis
see Stomach flu

Gastroenteritis

This is the general term for infections in the digestive tract. Variants are:

Diarrhea	*see* Diarrhea
Dysentery	*see* Dysentery
Food poisoning	*see* Food poisoning
Gastritis	*see* Stomach flu
Stomach flu	*see* Stomach flu
Traveler's diarrhea	*see* Diarrhea

Gastrointestinal Cleansing Formula
see GI Cleansing Formula

Gastrointestinal pain
see Stomachache

Legend: Preferred, Suggested, Consider

Genital herpes *(HHV-2)*

Oils: Lemongrass[C], Melaleuca[C], Melissa[EC]

1-2 drops Melissa or Lemongrass to outbreak area every 2 hours (not less than 3x daily). Continue for 3 days after symptoms are gone. For any of the oils and particularly Melissa dilution is recommended.

Additional protection: 1-2 drops Melissa in capsule 3x daily.

Strengthen immune system and emotions: Massage Blend Technique.

Reduce toxins: GI Cleansing Formula/Probiotic Defense Formula and/or Detoxification Blend cleansing.

Other oils: Frankincense[C]/Sandalwood[C] or Lavender[EC], Lemon[EC], Peppermint[C] **Blends/Products:** Detoxification Blend, Detoxification Complex, GI Cleansing Formula/Probiotic Defense Formula, Massage Blend, Protective Blend[C]

Genital warts   *see also* Warts

Oils: Frankincense[C], Melaleuca[C] **Blends:** Protective Blend[C]

2-3 drops Protective Blend or Melaleuca/Frankincense topically 2-3x daily. Usually requires 2-4 weeks, continue a week after gone. A carrier oil may facilitate application. For women soak end of tampon and use for internal genital warts.

Other oils: Oregano[C], Thyme[C]

Geranium *(Pelagronium graveolens)*

Properties: Analgesic, antidepressant, antiseptic, astringent, disinfectant, diuretic, sedative

Addresses: Acne, burns, cuts and wounds, depression, dermatitis, diarrhea, gum/mouth problems, herpes, hormone support, indigestion, menstrual problems, skin disorders, sore throat, stomachache, stress, throat infections

GERD   *see* Heartburn

German measles *(rubella)*   *see also* Measles

Oils: Eucalyptus, Lavender[c], Melaleuca[c]

Lavender topically to relieve symptoms of rash. Eucalyptus and Melaleuca internally to minimize the viral infection.

Other oils: Coriander **Blends:** Protective Blend

Germs   *see* Infections

GI Cleansing Formula *(Gastrointestinal)*

Product

Ingredients: Lemon, Lemongrass, Melaleuca, Oregano, Peppermint, Thyme and Caprylic acid.

This is a combination of essential oils and caprylic acid in softgel capsules that helps support a healthy digestive tract by creating an unfriendly environment for potentially harmful pathogens that can disrupt digestive immunities and cause digestive upset.

Giardia   *see* Food poisoning

Ginger *(Zingberaceae officinale)*

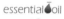

Properties: Analgesic, expectorant, stimulant

Addresses: Cold and flu, colic, congestion, constipation, diarrhea, fever, headaches, menstrual problems, motion sickness, muscle pain, nausea, sore throat, stomachache, throat infections

(see Safety Chart, page 23)

Gingivitis   *see* Gum conditions

Glaucoma   *see* Eyesight failing

Gluten intolerance   see Celiac disease

Gnats   *see* Insect repellent

Goiter

A goiter is the result of one of a number of thyroid conditions. Look to the links below for helpful suggestions. If you do not know the underlying condition search online based on the symptoms for clarification.

Graves' disease	*see* Hyperthyroidism
Hashimoto's disease	*see* Hypothyroidism
Hyperthyroidism	*see* Hyperthyroidism
Hypothyroidism	*see* Hypothyroidism
Thyroid nodules	*see* Thyroid nodules

Gout

Oils: Basil[EC], Frankincense, Lemon[EC] **Blends/Products:** Detoxification Blend/Detoxification Complex

Pain relief: 2-3 drops each Basil and Frankincense to area. After application cover with hot towel compress. Repeat 2-3 times daily (if area too sensitive to rub on oils make blend with water in spray bottle for application).

Other oils combinations using same procedure: Lemongrass/Wintergreen, or single oils: Basil, Peppermint or Soothing Blend.

Long term: Detoxification Blend/Detoxification Complex, 2-4 drops Lemon in glass of water 2-3x daily.

Other oils: Copaiba[C], Lemongrass, Peppermint, Wintergreen[C], Yarrow[C]

Blends: Soothing Blend[C]

GRAS

Definition A United States Food and Drug Administration (FDA) acronym for the phrase **G**enerally **R**ecognized **A**s **S**afe. The FDA requires this approval to food additives (substances that may be added to foods and taken internally). Products with this label must have a well documented history of safe use. Many essentials oils are GRAS, some are not. To be assured of safe internal use the product should have the GRAS notation on its packaging.

Grapefruit *(Citrus x paradisis)*

essential oil

Properties: Antidepressant, antiseptic, disinfectant, diuretic

Addresses: Acne, cold and flu, constipation, depression, skin conditions, weight loss

(see Safety Chart, page 23)

Graves' disease   *see* Hyperthyroidism

Green Mandarin *(Citrus nobilis or Citrus reticulata)*

essential oil

Properties: Antidepressant, antifungal, antioxidant, antiseptic, antispasmodic, calming, digestive, disinfectant, sedative, stimulant (digestive)

Addresses: Bacterial infections, calming (children), coughs, cuts & wounds, insomnia, poor circulation, poor digestion, stomachaches (children, elderly), stretch marks

(see Safety Chart, page 23)

Green Smoothie   *see also* **Fruit and Veggie Drink Mix**

Definition A nutritional supplement made with natural raw fruits and vegetables in a blender. A number of different recipes are online for different nutritional emphasis.

Grief   *see* Emotional strength

Grinding teeth   *see* Teeth grinding

Grounding Blend *(a life balancing help)*

essential oils
Blend

Ingredients: Blue Chamomile flower, Blue Tansy flower, Frankincense, Ho Wood, Spruce needle/leaf in a base of Fractionated Coconut Oil

Other common formulations: Angelica, Cedarwood, Juniper, Pine, Spruce, White fir, Ylang Ylang

And: Blue Tansy, Frankincense, Rosewood, Spruce in a base of almond oil

Addresses: Anxiety, attention deficit, hyperactivity, nervousness
(see Safety Chart, page 23)

Grounding Blend for Children   *see* Kid's Blends

Growing pains

Blends/Products: Basic Vitality Supplements, Chewable Multivitamins, Massage Blend, Omega-3 Fish Oil, Soothing Blend, Tension Blend

Pain: 2-3 drops Massage Blend, Soothing Blend or Tension Blend topically with light massage to painful area. Some have better success with one than another, experiment to find most effective for your child.

Help relax: Lavender or Roman Chamomile topically or to help sleep diffuse or put Lavender on pillow.

Nutrition: Chewable Multivitamins, Omega-3 Fish Oil, Basic Vitality Supplements

Other oils: Lavender, Lemon^C, Lemongrass, Peppermint, Roman Chamomile

Gum conditions   *see also* Oral hygiene, Teeth conditions

[Gingivitis (periodontal disease), Plaque]

Oils: Clove^C, Myrrh^{EC} **Blends/Products:** Protective Blend^C, Protective Blend Toothpaste

Pain: 1-2 drops Clove to area (dilute for children) **Reduce inflammation, short term help and gum health:**

Mild: 1-4 drops Protective Blend in Tbsp water or carrier oil. Swish and pull mixture through teeth for 5-10 minutes 2-3x daily, do not swallow. Add Lemon or Peppermint to improve taste. Follow by brushing with Protective Blend or Protective Blend Toothpaste. Other oils in place of Protective Blend include Melaleuca or Myrhh.

More aggressive: 2 Tbsp FCO with 2 drops each Clove and Oregano. Same procedure as above.

Abrasions: 1-4 drops Lavender or Melaleuca in Tbsp water or carrier oil. Swish and pull mixture through teeth for 5-10 minutes 2-3x daily. Do not swallow.

Simple sores: 1-2 drops Lavender or Melaleuca directly on sore.

Other oils: Lavender[C], Lemon[E], Melaleuca[C], Oregano

Notes:

Legend: Preferred, Suggested, Consider

H. pylori
see Ulcers

H1N1 (swine flu)
see Flu

Hair care
see also Baldness, Dandruff

[Dry, Fragile, Oily]

Oils: Clary Sage[C], Lavender[C], Lemon[C], Peppermint, Rosemary[C] **Blends/ Products:** Basic Vitality Supplements, Salon Essentials Protecting Shampoo, Smoothing Conditioner and Root to Tip Serum

Basic Vitality Supplements for strong and healthy hair.

Regular routine: Shampoo with A Protecting Shampoo, add 1-2 drops Rosemary to slow hair loss. Condition with A Smoothing Conditioner and an essential oil based Serum and/or add oils based on condition of hair then let conditioner remain for 2-3 minutes, rinse.

>   **Dry hair:** add 1-2 drops FCO plus 1-2 drops Lavender

>   **Oily hair:** add 1-2 drops Lemon and only use on tips and/or outer half of hair shaft

>   **Fragile hair:** add 1-2 drops Clary Sage

Before drying, spray with 2 oz water with 4 drops Peppermint or other oil, especially after color or perm.

Other oils: Basil, Geranium, Petitgrain[C], Roman Chamomile

Hair care (Essential oil based products)

Product

There are available a variety of healthy hair care products, some based on quality essential oils.

>   **Protecting Shampoo:** Based on Lime and Wild Orange essential oils with cleansers and plant extracts.

>   **Smoothing Conditioner:** Cedarwood, Eucalyptus, Lavandin, Lavender, Marjoram, Niaouli, Peppermint, Rosemary essential oils combined with conditioning emollients, botanical extracts and natural proteins.

Root to Tip Serum: Cedarwood, Eucalyptus, Lavandin, Lavender, Marjoram, Niaouli, Peppermint, Rosemary essential oils combined with nourishing lipids.

Healthy Hold Glaze: Protective and holding ingredients including Cedar wood, Eucalyptus, Lavandin, Lavender, Marjoram, Niaouli, Peppermint, Rosemary and Tangerine.

Hair conditions

Alopecia	*see* Baldness
Baldness	*see* Baldness
Dandruff	*see* Dandruff
Dry	*see* Hair care
Fragile	*see* Hair care
Loss	*see* Baldness
Oily	*see* Hair care
Stimulate growth	*see* Baldness

Hair loss
see Baldness

Halitosis
see Bad breath

Hand and Body lotions
see Personal care and Skin care

Hand-foot-mouth disease
[Coxsackievirus A16]

Oils: Eucalyptus, Lavender, Melaleuca **Blends:** Cleansing Blend, Protective Blend, Restful Blend

Reduce symptoms: 1 drop Protective Blend or Cleansing Blend with 1 tbsp FCO and apply to bottoms of feet and along spine 3-4 times daily.

For blisters and sores apply: 2 d Eucalyptus, 2 d Lavender mixed with 1 Tbsp FCO. When blisters pop apply 1 d Melaleuca, 1 d Lavender mixed with 1 Tbsp FCO. For mouth sores rub Protective Blend on end of finger directly on sores.

For calming: Restful Blend to back of neck.

Other Oils: Clove, Melissa **Blends:** Cellular Complex Blend

Legend: Preferred, Suggested, Consider

Hangovers

Oils: Lavender[C], Lemon[C], Rosemary[C]

2-3 drops each Lavender, Lemon and Rosemary in a warm bath.

Or make a blend of 1-2 drops each Grapefruit, Lavender, Lemon, Rosemary and Sandalwood blended with 1 Tbsp FCO. Massage blend on neck and back.

Other oils: Grapefruit[C], Sandalwood[C]

Hashimoto's thyroiditis   *see* Hypothyroidism

Hawaiian Sandalwood   *see Sandalwood*

Hay fever   *see* Allergies

Head injuries

[Coma, Concussion, Convulsions]

Oils: Frankincense[C], Helichrysum

1-2 drops Frankincense and Helichrysum 2x daily to bottom of brain stem and great toes. Basic Vitality Supplements daily is important. Massage Blend Technique often. Also 1-2 drops Frankincense under tongue daily.

Other oils: Bergamot[C], Cypress[C], Peppermint[C], Sandalwood[C] **Blends:** Grounding Blend[C]

Head lice   *see* Lice

Headache   *see also* Migraine headache

Oils: Frankincense[C], Lavender[EC], Peppermint[EC], Wintergreen[C] **Blends:** Tension Blend[C]

Mild tension headache: 1-2 drops Peppermint topically on temples, forehead and/or back of neck. Tension Blend topically also.

Sinus headaches: Tension Blend or Peppermint as above for immediate discomfort. Attend to sinus infection under Sinus Infections.

Severe headaches: Equal parts Frankincense, Lavender and Peppermint applied to temples, back of neck, crown of head and inhaled is highly recommended.

Another alternative is Peppermint or Tension Blend as described above, follow with damp, cool compress to forehead and/or back of neck. Inhaler or cup & inhale for added help. Rotate to Frankincense or Wintergreen oils if necessary.

For those with sensitive skin Peppermint and Wintergreen should be diluted with a carrier oil.

Other oils: Cardamom[EC], Copaiba[C], Cumin[C], Lemon[EC], Marjoram[EC], Neroli[C], Rosemary[EC], Spearmint, Yarrow[C] **Blends:** Soothing Blend[C]

Hearing loss

Oils: Geranium[C], Helichrysum[C], Lavender, White Fir **Blends:** Grounding Blend, Restful Blend

(Dr. Susan Lawton's protocol, see on YouTube) An abbreviated version:

Application technique: With each application apply the oils by first dripping them into palm of the receiving person and then the applying person dipping their finger in the oil and with a rubbing/massaging motion start at front of ear, then over fleshy rim of ear and down to lobe multiple times. Then follow down Eustachian tubes, starting at depression below and behind ears and down behind jaw line.

4 drops each Grounding Blend and Restful Blend and repeat the application technique above 10 times. 4 drops Helichrysum and repeat the application technique above 5 times. 2 drops each Lavender and White Fir and repeat the application technique 5 times. 3 drops Geranium and repeat the application technique 3 times.

Deeply inhale the mixture of oils that has accumulated in the palm of the hand. Gently pull and stretch the ear and surrounding area to stimulate the circulation and absorption of the oils that have been applied. Repeat this 2-3 times per week for 6-8 weeks.

Caution: Do not put oils directly into the ear.

Other oils: Eucalyptus[C], Fennel[E]

Legend: Preferred, Suggested, Consider

Heart conditions

[Arrhythmia (tachycarida), Arteriosclerosis, Atheriosclerosis, Atrial fibrillation, Cardiomyopathy, Congenital heart disease, Congestive heart failure, Coronary artery spasm, Coronary heart disease, Heart attack (myocardial infarction), Inflammatory heart disease, Palpitations, Pericarditis, Peripheral artery disease (PAD), Valvular heart disease]

Angina	*see* Angina
Cholesterol, high	*see* Cholesterol control
Circulation, poor	*see* Circulation, poor
High blood pressure	*see* Hypertension
Low blood pressure	*see* Hypotension

ATTENTION: If you are experiencing symptoms of heart attack

Call 911 immediately

Other suggestions commonly given:

Wait for ambulance., DO NOT DRIVE

Call someone to be with you

Take your prescribed nitroglycerin or chew an adult strength aspirin while waiting

Oils: Basil, Cypress[E], Frankincense, Ginger[C], Helichrysum, Lavender[EC], Lemon[C], Marjoram[C], Peppermint[EC], Rosemary[EC], Thyme[C], Wild Orange[EC], Ylang Ylang[EC] **Blends/Products:** Basic Vitality Supplements, Massage Blend

Heart conditions, as with many other serious health issues, should have treatment that includes professional medical attention.

Consistently use Basic Vitality Supplements and the Massage Blend Technique spinal treatment.

Blend equal parts Cypress, Helichrysum, Lavender and Marjoram and apply topically over heart, bottoms of feet and wrists at least 2x daily.

Or 3 drops each Lavender, Lemon, Marjoram, Ylang Ylang in capsule daily.

Supplement with oils from list below for specific needs:

Increases circulation: Peppermint

Improves circulation, reduce blood viscosity: Helichrysum

Balance heart function: Ylang Ylang

Help smooth muscle tissue (heart): Marjoram

Settle spasms: Cypress and Wild Orange

Settle arrhythmia symptoms: Soothing Blend, Lavender and Ylang Ylang

Arteriosclerosis circulation damage: Ginger, Lemon, Rosemary and Thyme

Settle increased heart rate: Lavender, Wild Orange and Ylang Ylang

Settle palpitations: Melissa, Peppermint and Ylang Ylang

Other oils: Geranium, Melissa[EC], Neroli[EC], Wintergreen[C] **Blends:** Protective Blend, Soothing Blend[C]

Heartburn (Acid reflux, GERD)

Oils: Cardamom[EC], Ginger[C], Peppermint[C], Sandalwood[C] **Blends:** Digestive Blend[C]

2-3 drops Ginger in mouthful of water (use shot glass), drink. Digestive Blend taken internally in a capsule, add Ginger. Peppermint or Wild Orange to strengthen, Frankincense topically on throat and chest, 3-5 drops Lemon in back of mouth, follow with water.

For infants: Digestive Blend with FCO rubbed on feet, stomach or chest (protect from baby touching area and rubbing eyes).

Other oils: Basil[EC], Black Pepper[E], Coriander[C], Eucalyptus[C], Frankincense, Lemon[C], Roman Chamomile[C], Wild Orange[C]

Heat exhaustion

[Dehydration, Heat stroke (Sun stroke)]

Oils: Peppermint[C]

Move to cool, restful position and hydrate by sipping cool liquids while applying oils:

2-5 drops Peppermint on cool damp cloth to forehead. (Sponge bath or body bath if extreme body temperature rise.) 2-3 drops Peppermint to each 1) back of neck 2) bottoms of feet 3) chest or neck. Use Peppermint spritz if available. Use cup & inhale with Peppermint.

Other oils: Lavender[EC]

Legend: Preferred, Suggested, Consider

| **Heat stroke** | *see* Heat exhaustion |

| **Heavy metals** | *see* Detoxification |

| **Heel pain** | *see* Bone spurs, Plantar fasciitis |

Helichrysum *(Helichrysum Italicum)*

essential oil

Properties: Analgesic, antifungal, anti-inflammatory, antioxidant, antiseptic, antispasmodic, astringent, disinfectant

Addresses: Arthritis, back pain, bruises and swelling, cuts and wounds, hypertension, insect bites, joint pain, nerve tissue, rosacea, scarring, skin care, sprains, stress

| **Hematoma** | *see* Bruise |

Hemorrhage *(bleeding)*

Also refer to pages on specific type of bleeding (a partial list):
> *Aneurysm*
> *Bruise and hematoma*
> *Cuts and wounds*
> *Hemorrhoids*
> *Nosebleed*
> *Pregnancy*
> *Stroke*

Oils: Frankincense[EC], Geranium[EC], Helichrysum[C], Rose[EC]

Minor hemorrhaging: 2-4 drops (more for large areas) topically to wound repeat as needed. Apply pressure manually or with a binding cloth to assist. Consider dangers of infection after stopping the bleeding.

Major hemorrhaging: Seek immediate professional medical help.

Other oils: Cinnamon Bark[E], Cypress[E], Eucalyptus[E], Ylang Ylang[C]

Hemorrhoids

Oils: Cypress[EC], Frankincense[EC], Helichrysum[EC], Lavender[C]

Mild/itching: 1-2 drops Helichrysum and/or Lavender directly to area of discomfort.

Bad/pain/itching: 1-2 drops Helichrysum, Frankincense and Lavender (or Cypress, Helichrysum and Lavender) directly to area of discomfort. Also use a cotton ball or other such material with 2-3 drops Frankincense as last wipe after bowel movements.

Internal: 1-2 drops each Geranium and Lavender (or blends above) with 1 tsp FCO internally as a rectal enema 3x daily until relieved.

Very bad/with bleeding: Use this blend: 2 Tbsp VCO, 10 drops each Cypress, Frankincense, Helichrysum, Lavender, 5 drops each Geranium and Sandalwood. 4-6 drops directly to area of discomfort 3x daily. Also use cotton ball or other such material with 2-3 drops Frankincense as the last wipe after bowel movements.

Additional comfort with all the above: Sitz baths, warm water in tub to cover hips with 2 -3 drops of oils.

Other oils: Geranium[C], Neroli[C], Peppermint, Sandalwood[C], Spikenard, Yarrow[C]

Hepatitis

Oils: Cilantro[C], Frankincense[C], Melissa **Blends/Products:** Basic Vitality Supplements, Detoxification Blend, Detoxification Complex, Protective Blend

Basic Vitality Supplements, Detoxification Complex tablets daily, 3-5 drops Detoxification Blend over liver area daily, 1 drop each Melissa and Protective Blend on thumb then transferred to roof of mouth 2x daily. Also consider using Cilantro with Oil Pulling daily.

Additional help: Grounding Blend or other oils/blends to relieve anxiety and stress, periodic use of the Massage Blend Technique, Soothing Blend Rub for pain relief.

Other oils: Basil[C], Cinnamon Bark[C], Geranium, Helichrysum, Melaleuca[C], Myrrh[C], Oregano[C], Ravensara[C], Rosemary[C], Thyme[C] **Blends:** Grounding Blend

Legend: Preferred, Suggested, Consider

Hernia

[Epigastric, Hiatal, Incisional, Inguinal, Umbilical]

Essential oils can be of help prior to surgery to help manage pain and after surgery to both manage pain, help speed up healing and be helpful to reduce scarring. Soothing Blend is good for deep muscle pain and will be helpful for most types of hernia pain as well as after surgery. Other oils are referenced below. All may be applied topically directly in the area of interest, use carrier oil if sensitive. A summary:

Encourage tissue repair (minor hernia or after surgery): Helichrysum[C], Frankincense, Lemongrass[C], Anti-Aging Blend[C]

Pain: Frankincense, Peppermint[C], Massage Blend, Soothing Blend

Acid reflux (hiatal hernia): Frankincense, Digestive Blend

Scar reduction: Helichrysum[C], Frankincense, Lavender[C]

Apply topically to local area, use carrier oil if sensitive.

Other oils: Abdominal: Basil[C], Geranium[C] Hiatal: Fennel[C], Ginger[C]

Herniated disk *see* Back conditions

Herpes simplex *see* Cold sores, Genital herpes

Herxheimer reaction *see also* **Detoxification**

 Definition

Aggressive detoxification or addressing infections can release toxins from the body faster than the liver can process them in a normal way and may cause uncomfortable digestive tract or skin rash conditions. Slow detoxification or slow and reduce anti-infectious agents if such occurs.

HFMD *see* Hand-Foot-Mouth disease

Hiatal hernia *see* Hernia

Hiccups

Oils: Dill[C], Peppermint, Sandalwood[EC]

Adults: 3-5 drops Peppermint in 2-3 oz (mouthful) water, swallow, expect

Peppermint jolt and relief.

Milder or for children: 2 drops Dill, 4 drops FCO, apply along lower edge of jaw line from base of earlobe, drink warm water slowly.

Other oils: Basil[E], Fennel[E], Tangerine[C]

High blood presssure
see Hypertension

HIV
see AIDS

Hives

Oils: Basil, Myrrh **Blends/Products:** GI Cleansing Formula/Probiotic Defense Formula

Internal toxins: GI Cleansing Formula for 10 days, Probiotic Defense Formula for 5 days, once a month, *see also* Detoxification.

Mild: 2-3 drops Basil or Myrhh topically to area.

Difficult: Alternate 2-3 drops Helichrysum/Melaleuca with 2-3 drops Frankincense to the affected area. Day 1 every 2 hours, day 2 every 4 hours, thereafter 3-4x daily until 2 days beyond hives are gone. Additional help by applying same oils along spine.

Other oils: Coriander, Frankincense, Helichrysum, Lavender[C], Lemon, Melaleuca[C], Peppermint[C]

Hodgkin disease (Hodgkin lymphoma)
see Cancer

Honesty
see Emotional strength

Hormonal balance (female)

Hormonal imbalance can be the root cause of many health concerns including unusual menstrual periods, endometriosis, hot flashes, difficult menopause, PCOS and PMS.

General suggestions
Basic Vitality Supplements, Monthly Blend for Women, Phytoestrogen Complex

Consistent Basic Vitality Supplements and Phytoestrogen Complex

(Perimenopausal 1-2 capsules daily with food. Post-menopausal 2 capsules daily with food.) 1-2 drops Monthly Blend for Women bottoms of feet, back of neck, temples or inhale.

Reduce stress

Bergamot[C], Frankincense[C], Massage Blend, Roman Chamomile[C], Sandalwood[C]

2-3 drops Sandalwood or 1 drop each Bergamot, Frankincense and Roman Chamomile mixed together. Apply to the bottoms of feet, back of neck, temples and/or inhale the aroma.

The Massage Blend Technique twice a month at least, more often if needed.

Control toxicity

Basic Vitality Supplements, Detoxification Blend/ Detoxification Complex, GI Cleansing Formula/Probiotic Defense Formula, Lemon[C]

Basic Vitality Supplements, Detoxification Blend cleanse (see Detoxification), GI Cleansing Formula/Probiotic Defense Formula (see Detoxification), add 2-5 drops Lemon or other citrus oil per glass of water or 10-15 drops in capsule daily.

Decrease adrenaline

Blend for Women[C], Patchouli, Rose

Increase natural progesterone

Frankincense[C], Geranium[C], Oregano[C], Thyme[C]

Use natural sources, Basic Vitality Supplements, 1-2 drops Thyme and/or Oregano to bottoms of feet (limit Oregano to 8-10 days). Geranium topically over liver, adrenal glands and/or kidneys.

Symptoms

Hot flashes: Citrus oils, Clary Sage[C], Geranium[C], Grounding Blend[C], Monthly Blend for Women[C], Peppermint[C]

Peppermint on feet at night, back of neck, chest or spray bottle with Peppermint and water. Others prefer or use Monthly Blend for Women additionally applied to inside of ankles.

Fatigue: Basic Vitality Supplements, Energy & Stamina Complex,

Ginger, Peppermint, White Fir

Oils inhaled or on temples, Ginger topically to liver and adrenal glands. Basic Vitality Supplements and Energy & Stamina Complex.

Insomnia: Restful Blend^C, Lavender, Roman Chamomile^C, Spikenard^C

Inhale or put on pillow at night.

Libido: Clary Sage^C, Ginger, Joyful Blend^C, Peppermint, Ylang Ylang^C

Diffuse or use as perfume.

Memory loss: Frankincense, Peppermint, Rosemary

Diffuse or apply to temples and back of neck.

Other oils: Clary Sage^C, Grapefruit^C, Lime^C, Spikenard^C, Ylang Ylang^C, Yarrow^C **Blends:** Blend for Women^C, Grounding Blend^C, Joyful Blend^C, Restful Blend^C

Hormonal balance (male)

Oils: Clary Sage^C, Fennel^C, Frankincense^C, Ylang Ylang^C

1-2 drops each Clary Sage, Frankincese and Ylang Ylang topically to lower abdomen, reflexology points on feet and/or in capsule daily. Consider other oil combinations.

Other oils: Geranium^C, Ginger^C, Rosemary^C **Blends:** Blend for Women

Horse care

Oils suggestions from others:

Cuts and wounds: Lavender, Melaleuca, Protective Blend

Focus: Basil, Cypress

Fracture: Ginger with hot compress

Hoof rot: 1 drop each Melissa, Roman Chamomile, Thyme, 1 Tbsp FCO, apply topically

Infection (bacterial, fungal): Lavender, Melaleuca, Protective Blend

Insect repellent: Peppermint, Repellent Blend

Legend: Preferred, Suggested, Consider

Muscle strain: Lavender, Lemongrass with FCO and wrap

Nervous: Grounding Blend, Restful Blend, Lavender, Frankincense

Physical disorders: Mix 1-2 drops essential oils with FCO and apply topically. Repeat often.

Emotional disorders: Rub 1-2 drops on hands and cup under horse's nose or rub on the ears. Do not force.

Hot flashes   *see also* Hormonal balance

Oils: Clary Sage[C], Geranium[C], Peppermint[C], Ylang Ylang **Blends:** Blend for Women, Grounding Blend[C], Monthly Blend for Women[C]

Immediate symptoms: Peppermint on back of neck, chest, feet at night or spray bottle with Peppermint and water.

Extreme discomfort: Blend for Women and Ylang Ylang on back of neck and/or ears morning and night. Others prefer or use Monthly Blend for Women applied to ankles.

On going: Grounding Blend, Clary Sage and Peppermint on back of neck in morning, Geranium and Peppermint during day as needed.

Root cause: *see* Hormonal balance

Other oils: Citrus Oils[C], Lavender[C]

Household care

Air freshener

Diffuse a selected essential oil:
Pleasant atmosphere: Invigorating Blend, Wild Orange or your favorite oil
Basic disinfecting: Cleansing Blend, Lemon, Protective Blend
Mood enhancement: Joyful Blend, Lavender, Restful Blend
Congestion: Eucalyptus, Respiratory Blend
Insomnia: Restful Blend, Lavender

Air quality   *see* Air quality

Ants *(small black kitchen ants)*

Oils: Lemongrass, Peppermint

Keep counters clear of food and spills, especially overnight. Combine 20 drops Lemongrass, ¼ - ½ cup grapeseed oil in spray bottle. Shake well and often. Spray areas where ants commonly enter or congregate, then wipe down.

Bathroom cleaning

Oils: Lemon **Blends:** Protective Blend, Protective Blend Cleaner Concentrate

Protective Blend Cleaner Concentrate, follow directions on bottle or mix in 1 quart of clean hot water, 1 cup white vinegar, 1 Tbsp natural soap, 20 drops Protective Blend, 10 drops Lemon and use generously.

Bed freshener

Blends: Invigorating Blend

½-1 cup distilled water, 10-20 drops Invigorating Blend in spray bottle. Spray to freshen bed linens as bed is made or prior to bedtime. Also a few drops Eucalyptus occasionally for dust mites and use Lavender or Restful Blend to help induce restful sleep.

Carpet refreshing

Oils: Lavender, Lemon, Oregano, Peppermint **Blends:** Blend for Women, Restful Blend, Invigorating Blend, Joyful Blend, Protective Blend

Make a shaker with empty "Pringles" type canister with small holes punched in plastic lid with hole punch. Mix 15-20 drops essential oils of choice from below with 1 box baking soda and add to shaker. Sprinkle onto carpet, let sit, then vacuum. Choose one of following:

10 drops Lavender, 5 drops each Lemon and Oregano

20 drops Protective Blend

20 drops Joyful Blend, Blend for Women or Restful Blend to set a mood.

10 drops each Invigorating Blend and Peppermint

Closet and drawer freshener

Blends: Invigorating Blend

Legend: Preferred, Suggested, Consider

½-1 cup distilled water, 10-20 drops Invigorating Blend or other pleasing oils in spray bottle, spray closet or drawers to freshen them.

Countertop disinfectant

Blends: Cleansing Blend, Protective Blend, Protective Blend Cleaner Concentrate

Protective Blend Cleaner Concentrate, follow directions on bottle. Or fill spray trigger bottle with 1 cup each distilled white vinegar and distilled water, 35 drops Protective Blend, 5 drops Cleansing Blend and shake to mix well. Spray on countertops, shake often. Other oil combinations:

30 drops Melaleuca, 5 drops each Lavender and Peppermint

30 drops White Fir, 5 drops each Grapefruit and Melaleuca

Deodorizing areas   *see* Deodorizing areas

Dishwasher, cleaning

Oils: Lemon

Add 4-5 drops of Lemon in a small bowl of water in the dishwasher and run as a normal load.

Dishwashing soap, homemade

Oils: Lavender, Lemon, Melaleuca, Peppermint, Wild Orange
Blends: Invigorating Blend, Protective Blend

Grate 1 Tbsp castile soap and place in mixing bowl with 1 Tbsp borax, add 1 3/4 cup hot water and stir until dissolved, let cool, add 15-20 drops essential oils and mix thoroughly. Try Invigorating Blend, Lavender, Lemon, Melaleuca, Protective Blend, Peppermint, Wild Orange or your favorite oil.

Dishwashing soap, simple

Oils: Lavender, Lemon, Melaleuca, Peppermint, White Fir, Wild Orange **Blends:** Invigorating Blend, Protective Blend

Add several drops of Invigorating Blend to commercial dishwashing soap with each dishwasher load. Also try Lavender, Lemon, Melaleuca, Protective Blend, Peppermint, White Fir or Wild Orange.

Fruit and vegetable cleaning

Oils: Lemon, Wild Orange **Blends:** Invigorating Blend, Protective Blend

5-20 drops Lemon, Wild Orange, Invigorating Blend or Protective Blend in sink with water. Place fruits or vegetables in colander, lower into water and agitate, then dry.

Furniture polish

Oils: Lemon **Blends:** Invigorating Blend, Wild Orange

30 drops Lemon, 1/3 cup FCO, 1/2 cup distilled water, 10 drops Wild Orange or Invigorating Blend (optional) combined in spray trigger bottle and shake to mix well. Spray on furniture, wipe with soft cloth, shake often.

Hard floor cleaning

Oils: Lemon **Blends:** Cleansing Blend, Protective Blend, Protective Blend Cleaner Concentrate

Protective Blend Cleaner Concentrate, follow directions on bottle. Or add 1/4 cup white vinegar, 3-10 drops dishwashing soap, 5-10 drops Protective Blend, Cleansing Blend and/or Lemon to bucket (about 1 gallon) of warm filtered water.

Laundry, dryer

Oils: Lavender, Lemon, Melaleuca **Blends:** Invigorating Blend

Place washcloth dampened with 10 drops of Lavender, Lemon, Melaleuca, Invigorating Blend or another essential oil you enjoy. While the oils will not reduce static cling, they will impart a distinctive fragrance to your clothes.

Laundry, homemade fabric softener

Oils: Lavender **Blends:** Invigorating Blend

Mix 6 cups water, 1/2 cup baking soda. Slowly add 3 cups white vinegar and allow chemical interaction. Then add 10-20 drops Invigorating Blend, Lavender or favorite oil. Use one cup of softener in final rinse cycle.

Laundry, washing with commercial soap

Oils: Eucalyptus, Lavender, Lemon **Blends:** Invigorating Blend, Protective Blend Laundry Detergent

10 drops each Lemon (deodorize/sanitize) and Eucalyptus (dust mites/fleas) added to cycle with commercial soap (preferably non-perfumed soap). 2-10 drops of Invigorating Blend, Lavender or Lemon to rinse cycle to further soften and deodorize.

Laundry, washing with homemade soap

Oils: Eucalyptus, Lavender, Lemon **Blends:** Invigorating Blend

Stir together 1 bar castile soap shaved, 1 cup borax (20 Mule Team) and 1 cup washing soda (Arm & Hammer) for homemade soap. Then add 10 drops each Lemon (deodorize/sanitize) and Eucalyptus (dust mites/fleas) with 1-2 Tbsp homemade soap for wash cycle. 2-10 drops of Invigorating Blend, Lavender or Lemon to rinse cycle to further soften and deodorize.

Mildew   *see* Mold and mildew

Mold   *see* Mold and mildew

Painting, headache

Oils: Peppermint **Blends:** Soothing Blend, Tension Blend

1-2 drops Tension Blend or Peppermint to temples, forehead or back of neck.

Painting, improve odor

Oils: Lemon, Peppermint, Wild Orange **Blends:** Invigorating Blend

10-30 drops per gallon Invigorating Blend, Lemon, Peppermint, Wild Orange to add pleasant odor. Also consider Grounding Blend, Joyful Blend, Geranium, Grapefruit, Lime, Rosemary, Restful Blend.

Painting, reduce fumes

Oils: Peppermint **Blends:** Cleansing Blend

50-100 drops Peppermint, Cleansing Blend or other favorite smelling oil per gallon paint.

Toilet bowl cleaner

Oils: Melaleuca **Blends:** Protective Blend

Mix 1 cup white vinegar and 5-10 drops Protective Blend or Melaleuca in spray bottle, spray inside bowl. Mix 1 cup baking soda and 1/4 cup salt and sprinkle on vinegar mixture. Let stand 10-15 minutes, scrub with brush and flush.

Vacuum cleaner

Drip several drops of favorite oils on tissue and place in collection bag of vacuum. This will diffuse pleasant odor as you clean as well as reduce airborne microbes.

Vents, AC/heater

Oils: Cassia, Oregano, Peppermint **Blends:** Cleansing Blend, Invigorating Blend, Protective Blend

Change air return filters often, add 10 drops of favorite oil to reduce pathogens. Consider Protective Blend, Invigorating Blend, Cleansing Blend, Oregano, Peppermint or Cassia.

Water purification

see Water purification

Window and mirror cleaning

Oils: Lemon, Wild Orange

10-15 drops Lemon or Wild Orange added to 1 cup each white vinegar and filtered water in spray bottle. Shake well before using, spray, wipe and buff with paper towel or newspaper.

Household care products

Product

Products for household care based on essential oils are available.

Protective Blend Laundry Detergent: Amazing clean clothes with a ultra-concentrated laundrydetergent.

Protective Blend Cleaner Concentrate: A natural cleaner for all hard surfaces in the home.

Legend: Preferred, Suggested, Consider

Human immunodeficiency virus *see* AIDS

Huntington's disease

Oils: Frankincense[C], Helichrysum, Rosemary, Ylang Ylang[C] **Blends/Products:** Basic Vitality Supplements, Grounding Blend, Joyful Blend, Massage Blend, Restful Blend

Basic Vitality Supplements and 2 drops Frankincense under the tongue daily.

Apply one or more of oils above to meridian points, crown of head, base of the skull, etc. at least daily. Experiment to minimize symptoms and help with emotional ups and downs. Some suggest rotating oils.

Other oils: Clary Sage, Clove, Oregano

Hydrating skin *see* Personal care and Skin care

Hydrocarbons *see* Chemical constituents

Hyperactivity *see* ADD/ADHD

Hyperglycemia *see* Diabetes

Hypertension *(high blood pressure)*

Oils: Basil[C], Clary Sage[EC], Lavender[EC], Marjoram[EC], Ylang Ylang[EC] **Blends/Products:** Basic Vitality Supplements

Serious circulatory conditions, as with many other health issues, are best treated with professional medical attention.

Recommendations: 1) make positive dietary changes 2) exercise daily 3) use Basic Vitality Supplements daily 4) use reduced amount of quality sea salt 5) find essential oils that are effective at reducing your blood pressure.

Consider massage 2-4 drops oil or blend to bottoms of feet, wrists, breast bone, over heart, on carotidal arteries and back of neck. Choose oil from those recommended above (or below) using muscle testing, inhaling various oils and using impression or instinct. If unsure, the most highly recommended are Clary Sage, Lavender, Marjoram and Ylang Ylang.

This is a serious condition and if control is not achieved seek professional medical help.

The following is the success of one person with stage 2 hypertension and their comments; 3 drops each Basil, Lavender, Marjoram in a capsule daily. Each person is different and may respond to other oils. This will take testing and patience. Try a new oil or blend, take BP before and after in varying intervals, 5 min, 1 hr, 8 hrs and 16 hrs. Try applying oils hourly, every 8 hrs and every 24 hours. Keep a record of results.

Other oils: Cassia, Frankincense, Helichrysum, Lemon[EC], Neroli[C], Yarrow[C] **Blends:** Invigorating Blend[C], Restful Blend[C]

Hypertensive heart disease   *see* Hypertension

Hyperthyroidism   *see also* Autoimmune diseases

Oils: Frankincense[C], Lemongrass[C], Myrrh[C]

GI Cleansing Formula/Probiotic Defense Formula detoxification (*see* Detoxification), Basic Vitality Supplements, 2-3 drops each Lemongrass (dilute with carrier if skin sensitivity) and Myrrh topically to thyroid area, reflexology points on feet (big toes) and on wrists multiple times daily. 2 drops Frankincense under tongue daily.

For symptoms:

Pain: Soothing Blend Rub to thyroid area.

Tiredness and depression: Joyful Blend, citrus oils, Peppermint. Diffuse or cup and inhale.

Anxiety and irritability: Grounding Blend and Melissa. Diffuse or cup and inhale.

Other oils: Melissa[C] **Blends:** Soothing Blend

Hypochromic anemia   *see* Anemia

Hypoglycemia   *see* Diabetes

Legend: Preferred, Suggested, Consider

Hypotension *(low blood pressure)*

Oils: Cypress, Geranium[C], Rosemary[EC] **Blends:** Restful Blend

Blend 2 parts Rosemary and 1 part each Geranium and Cypress with 4 parts carrier oil and apply to chest and bottoms of feet. Also consider diffusion periodically.

Other oils: Blue Tansy, Helichrysum[C], Lemon[C], Lime[C], Peppermint, Rose[C], Thyme[EC]

Hypothermia

Oils: Lavender **Blends:** Grounding Blend, Invigorating Blend

This should be considered a life threatening medical emergency. Seek professional medical attention. Interim procedures would include warming the individual but not too rapidly (1 degree F/hour recommended). After stable use oils to relax and calm.

Hypothyroidism   *see also* Autoimmune diseases
[Hashimoto's disease]

Oils: Frankincense, Geranium, Lemongrass[C], Myrrh[C] **Blends:** Grounding Blend

GI Cleansing Formula/Probiotic Defense Formula detoxification, Basic Vitality Supplements, 2-4 drops Grounding Blend and Geranium, 2-4 drops Lemongrass and Myrrh. Alternate two combinations weekly, topically to thyroid area, reflexology points on feet (great toes) and on wrists multiple times daily. Supplement with Peppermint and Clove.

For symptoms:

Pain: Soothing Blend Rub to thyroid area.

Tiredness and depression: Joyful Blend, citrus oils, Peppermint. Diffuse or cup and inhale.

Anxiety and irritability: Grounding Blend and Melissa. Diffuse or cup and inhale.

Other oils: Clove[C], Melissa[C], Peppermint[C]

Hysteria   *see* Mood swings

Notes:

Legend: Preferred, Suggested, Consider

IBD
see Inflammatory bowel disease

IBS
see Irritable bowel syndrome

Impetigo
see also Ecthyma

Oils: Lavender^C, Melaleuca **Blends:** Protective Blend

2-3 drops Protective Blend with carrier oil to area 3-4x daily until infection gone plus 2-3 days. Also consider Lavender/Melaleuca if Protective Blend not available. Keep area dry and free of fluid from blister.

Use Protective Blend Foaming Hand Wash to cleanse caregiver as infection is highly contagious.

Myrrh^C **Blends/Products:** Cleansing Blend, Protective Blend Foaming Hand Wash

Impotence
see Aphrodisiac, Erectile dysfunction, Libido

Incisional hernia
see Hernia

Incontinence

Oils: Clove^C, Cypress^C, Frankincense^C, Lavender^C, Thyme^C **Blends:** Invigorating Blend^C

Female related incontinence: Apply and rub 2 -3 drops Cypress over bladder and also consider coupling with Kegel exercises.

Prostate related incontinence: Make blend of 5 parts each Frankincense and Invigorating Blend; 3 parts each Clove, Lavender and Thyme. Place 10-13 drops of this blend in capsule 2-3x daily.

Other oils: Copaiba^C

Indigestion

Oils: Fennel^E, Ginger^{EC}, Peppermint^{EC}, Roman Chamomile^{EC} **Blends:** Digestive Blend^C, GI Cleansing Formula/Probiotic Defense Formula

Children/Adults: 1-5 drops Digestive Blend. *(Ginger, Fennel, or Peppermint if Digestive Blend not available).* Internally in capsule or with water, juice, tsp of honey or agave. Or rub on abdomen with carrier if needed.

Chronic indigestion: 2-3 Digestive Enzyme Complex capsules and 2-3 drops Fennel in glass of water daily as well as a gastro-intestinal cleanse with GI Cleansing Formula/Probiotic Defense Formula (*see* Detoxification).

Small children/sensitive skin: Dilute with carrier and rub on tummy.

Very sensitive skin: Apply to bottoms of feet.

Infants: Apply a carrier oil on the tummy followed by 1-2 drops of Digestive Blend (or one of the other listed oils). Warm hands, massage baby's tummy and lower back with circular motions. Hold and cuddle baby close afterwards. Consider also applying a warm *(not hot)* compress or towel warmed in the dryer. Applying oils and carrier to feet with a foot massage is also effective.

Other oils: Basil[EC], Coriander[EC], Cumin[C], Dill[C], Frankincense[EC], Lavender[EC], Marjoram[EC], Myrrh[EC], Rosemary[EC], Spearmint[C], Spikenard[C], Star Anise[C]

Infant/toddler care

Baby dry skin	*see* Skin care, infants
Colic	*see* Colic
Cradle cap	*see* Skin care, infants
Crying	*see* Irritability, infants
Diaper rash	*see* Skin care, infants
Diarrhea	*see* Diarrhea
Jaundice	*see* Jaundice
Teething	*see* Teething
Tummy ache	*see* Indigestion

Consider these general suggestions:

> **Skin test:** It is suggested to use a skin test with each new oil to determine skin sensitivity. See Safety Considerations in the front of this book for information on skin testing.

Legend: Preferred, Suggested, Consider

Protect from transfer: If oils are applied to feet of infants it is recommended to cover with socks to prevent them from inadvertently transferring oils to their eyes.

Digestive problems: Apply a carrier oil on the tummy followed by blend or single oil (see specific condition above). With warm hands massage baby's tummy and lower back with circular motions. Hold and cuddle baby close afterwards. Consider also applying a warm (not hot) compress or towel warmed in the dryer. Applying oils and carrier to feet with a foot massage is also effective.

Infections

Bacterial	*see* Bacterial infections
Fungal	*see* Fungal infections
MRSA	*see* MRSA
Parasites	*see* Parasite infections
Staph	*see* Staph infections
Viral	*see* Viral infection

Infertility (female)

Blends/Products: Basic Vitality Supplements, GI Cleansing Formula/Probiotic Defense Formula

The most common recommendation is to do a candida cleanse using GI Cleansing Formula/Probiotic Defense Formula protocol at least monthly, it can be safely used on a monthly basis if needed. 1-3 GI Cleansing Formula capsules daily with meals for 10 days, followed with 1 capsule of Probiotic Defense Formula 3x daily with food for 5 days.

see also Candida and Detoxification for other suggestions.

Basic Vitality Supplements consistently.

Other oils: Clary Sage[C], Cypress[C], Fennel[C], Geranium[C], Thyme[C], Ylang Ylang[E]

Infertility (male)

Oils: Basil[C], Clary Sage[C], Thyme[C]

Clary Sage inhalation and topically for hormonal conditions, Basil and

Thyme, 3 drops 2x daily in a capsule for possible infections. Basic Vitality Supplements consistently. GI Cleansing Formula/Probiotic Defense Formula should be considered.

Inflammation

[Acute, Chronic]

Oils and blends below are those suggested by a noted essential oils expert for general inflammation concerns:

Basic Vitality Supplements, Frankincense, Helichrysum, Massage Blend, Myrrh

Basil, Eucalyptus, Ginger, Juniper Berry, Lavender, Peppermint, Siberian Fir[C], Wintergreen

Cassia, Cinnamon Bark, Clove, Geranium, Jasmine, Lemon, Oregano, Roman Chamomile, Thyme, Ylang Ylang

Also: Blue Tansy, Cilantro, Citrus Oils, Clary Sage, Copaiba[C], Coriander, Fennel, Lemongrass, Melaleuca, Melissa, Patchouli, Petitgrain, Rose, Sandalwood, Yarrow

Chronic inflammation: Basic Vitality Supplements and Massage Blend Technique periodically. See the specific chronic conditions.

Acute inflammation: See the specific conditions. Generally consider topical or internal use of one/some of the oils above.

Inflammatory bowel disease (colitis, IBD, ulcerative colitis)

see also Autoimmune diseases

Oils: Frankincense[C], Peppermint **Blends/Products:** Basic Vitality Supplements, Digestive Blend, Digestive Enzyme Complex, GI Cleansing Formula/Probiotic Defense Formula, Massage Blend

Symptom relief: 2-5 drops each Digestive Blend and Frankincense in capsule or 2-5 drops Digestive Blend or Peppermint topically to abdominal area.

Long term support: Basic Vitality Supplements, GI Cleansing Formula/Probiotic Defense Formula cleanse, periodic use of Massage Blend Technique.

Infectious IBD: 10 drops Thyme and Oregano, 4 drops Frankincense

Legend: Preferred, Suggested, Consider

with 35 drops coconut carrier oil. 10 drops of this blend in capsules. 2x daily with meals. Continue for 5 days after symptoms subside. Also daily Massage Blend Technique.

Other oils: Frankincense, Fennel, Ginger, Oregano, Thyme

Inflammatory heart disease
see Heart conditions

Influenza
see Flu

Inguinal hernia
see Hernia

Inhaler

 Definition A commercially available device similar to a Vicks inhaler except it is configured so you can add the oil or blend of your choice to an internal wick to make any "flavor" of inhaler you desire.

Insect bites
see also Insect repellent

Bed bugs	*see* Bed bugs
Bee stings	*see* Bee stings
Chiggers	*see* Chiggers
Fleas	*see* Fleas
Lice	*see* Lice
Mites	*see* Scabies
Mosquitoes	*see* Mosquito bites
Spiders	*see* Spider bites
Ticks	*see* Lyme disease
Wasps	*see* Bee stings
Yellow jackets	*see* Bee stings

Insect repellent
see also Insect bites

Ants: Lemongrass, Outdoor Blend, Peppermint, Rosemary
   Also consider: Eucalyptus, Lemon^E, Wild Orange
   see also Household care

Aphids: Peppermint

Beetles: Outdoor Blend

Also consider: Peppermint, Thyme

Chiggers: Lavender, Lemongrass, Outdoor Blend, Thyme

Cockroaches: Cypress[C]

Cutworm: Thyme

Fleas: Outdoor Blend
Also consider: Cleansing Blend, Lavender, Lemongrass, Peppermint

Gnats: Clove[EC], Eucalyptus[EC], Outdoor Blend
Also consider: Basil[C], Geranium[E], Lavender[C], Lemon[C], Lemongrass[C], Melaleuca[C], Peppermint[C], Thyme[C], Wild Orange[C]

Mites, dust: Basil[C], Eucalyptus[C], Lemongrass[C]

Mosquitoes: Outdoor Blend
Also consider: Basil[C], Cedarwood[EC], Clove[EC], Eucalyptus[EC], Geranium[E], Lavender[C], Lemongrass[C], Melaleuca[C], Peppermint[C], Thyme[C], Wild Orange[C]

Moths: Cedarwood[EC], Cleansing Blend, Clove[E], Lavender[E], Lemon[E], Peppermint, Repellent Blend

Plant Lice: Peppermint

Spiders: Cleansing Blend, Outdoor Blend, Peppermint

Ticks: Lavender, Lemongrass, Thyme, Cleansing Blend

Black Widow: Oregano

Scorpion: Basil

Insomnia

Oils: Clary Sage[C], Frankincense[C], Lavender[EC], Roman Chamomile[EC], Ylang Ylang[EC] **Blends:** Restful Blend[C]

2-3 drops of Lavender, Neroli or Restful Blend on hands and rubbed across pillow at bedtime. Or 1-3 drops Clary Sage under tongue at bedtime. 5% Lavender and water in spray bottle and spray pillow.

Experiment: Other oils or baths, body or foot massage, inhaling or diffusing at bedtime may provide a better personal response. A Massage Blend Technique at bedtime is a great relaxant.

Legend: Preferred, Suggested, Consider

Even after finding the best personal oil and application it may prove beneficial to rotate with other oils/application from time to time.

Children: Foot massage at bedtime using Restful Blend, Lavender or a blend of Lemon/Lavender/carrier oil.

Other oils: Bergamot^C, Green Mandarin^{EC}, Jasmine^C, Litsea^{EC}, Magnolia^C, Marjoram^{EC}, Neroli^{EC}, Petitgrain^{EC}, Sandalwood^{EC}, Spikenard^C, Star Anise^C, Wild Orange^{EC}

Inspiring Blend

(comes in a roll-on dispenser)

Ingredients: Cardamom, Cinnamon Bark, Clove, Damiana, FCO, Ginger, Jasmine, Sandalwood, Vanilla

Addresses: An emotional health blend to help strengthen enthusiasm, passion and zest

(see Safety Chart, page 23)

Interstitial cystitis   see UTI

Intestinal parasites   see Parasite infections

Invigorating Blend *(for bliss with energy)*

(also available in a Bath Bar and Hand Lotion)

Ingredients: Clementine peel, Grapefruit, Lemon, Mandarin peel, Tangerine peel, Vanilla bean absolute, Wild Orange

Another common formulation: Grapefruit, Lemon, Mandarin, Orange, Tangerine, Spearmint

Addresses: Calming, disinfects surfaces, elevating, eliminates odors, kills airborne pathogens, strengthens immune system

(see Safety Chart, page 23)

Iritis   see Eyesight failing

Iron deficiency   see Anemia

Irritability *(anger)*   *see also* Hormonal balance

Oils: Blue Tansy[C], Lavender[EC], Patchouli, Tangerine[C] **Blends:** Blend for Women, Grounding Blend, Restful Blend

Emotional balance: Grounding Blend, Blue Tansy, Lavender, Patchouli or Restful Blend topically to back of neck and/or cup & inhale or diffuse.

Headaches: Tension Blend to back of neck, temples or above eyebrows.

Sleep: Lavender, Neroli, Patchouli or Sandalwood or Restful Blend applied topically to bottoms of feet and/or diffuse while sleeping.

Infants: For crying see also suggestions under Infant care, Colic and Teething. Lavender or Restful Blend on bottoms of feet to soothe and relax.

Other oils: Bergamot[EC], Cedarwood[C], Clary Sage[C], Grapefruit, Magnolia[C], Melissa[EC], Myrrh[C], Petitgrain[EC], Roman Chamomile[EC], Rose[EC], Sandalwood[EC], Ylang Ylang[EC] **Blends:** Comforting Blend, Focus Blend, Joyful Blend, Renewing Blend, Tension Blend

Irritable bowel syndrome *(IBS)*

Oils: Ginger, Frankincense, Peppermint[C] **Blends/Products:** Basic Vitality Supplements, Digestive Blend[C], GI Cleansing Formula/Probiotic Defense Formula

Detoxify/fortify gut with GI Cleansing Formula/Probiotic Defense Formula, consistent Basic Vitality Supplements, Daily capsule of 5 drops Digestive Blend, 2 drops Ginger, 4 drops Frankincense.

Also research confirms 3-5 drops Peppermint in capsule 3x daily with fiber helps.

Other oils: Fennel, Geranium[C]

Itchy eye   *see* Eye injury or discomfort

    Legend: Preferred, Suggested, Consider

Itchy skin

Oils: Lavender[C], Melaleuca[C], Patchouli[C], Peppermint[EC] **Blends:** Cleansing Blend

Mild: 2-3 drops Lavender or Peppermint to area (dilute for larger areas or sensitive skin).

Severe: Add 2-3 drops Frankincense or Protective Blend.

Also consider the possibility of internal toxins, nutrition or stress, irritants in laundry or personal care products. Use non-toxic products, detoxification, diet, Restful Blend or Massage Blend Technique.

Other Oils: Blue Tansy[C], Frankincense, Neroli[EC], Roman Chamomile[E]
Other Blends/Products: GI Cleansing Formula/Probiotic Defense Formula, Protective Blend, Restful Blend

Notes:

Legend: Preferred, Suggested, Consider

Jasmine *(Jasminum grandiflorum)*

essential oil

(comes in a roll-on)

Properties: Analgesic, antibacterial, antidepressant, antispasmodic, aphrodisiac, calming, expectorant, sedative

Addresses: Anxiety, aphrodisiac, breast feeding (increase supply), colds, conjunctivitis, congestion, cough, cuts and wounds, depression, despair, eczema (emotional), emotional fatigue, fatigue (physical), headache, hormone balance, insomnia, laryngitis, libido (low men), libido (low women), menstrual cramps, mood swings, mucous, muscle cramps pain killer, postpartum depression, pregnancy (delivery preparation), pregnancy (early labor), pregnancy (labor), prostate conditions, scar reduction, sedative, spasmodic cough, skin (dry), skin (mature), skin (oily), skin (sensitive), skin (wrinkles), skin (stretch marks), snoring, sprains, stress

Note: Some point out that although Jasmine is effective for many things there are other oils that will address the same issues that are much less expensive. Commonly available Jasmine is an absolute oil.

(see Safety Chart, page 23)

Jaundice   *see also* Infant care

Oils: Geranium^C, Lemon^{EC}, Rosemary^C

Babies. 1-2 drops each Geranium and Lemon in palm of hand, gently rub bottoms of baby's feet.

Children/adults. Geranium and Lemon to bottoms of feet, topically over liver (with carrier if needed) and/or liver reflexology points.

Other oils: Clove^E, Eucalyptus^E, Frankincense, Lavender^E, Thyme^E

Jet lag

Oils: Geranium[C], Lavender[C], Peppermint[C], Rosemary[C] **Blends:** Joyful Blend[C], Focus Blend[C]

Healthy nutrition/hydrations: Basic Vitality Supplements and Lemon or Grapefruit in water, avoid alcohol, coffee and other artificial stimulants.

Relax: Grounding Blend or Lavender

Sleep at the right time: Lavender or Geranium inhale, diffuse, baths.

Alertness at the right time: Peppermint for alertness, Joyful Blend for energy, Focus Blend or Vetiver for focus.

Other oils: Eucalyptus[C], Grapefruit[C], Lemongrass[C] **Blends:** Grounding Blend[C]

Jock itch

Oils: Lavender[C], Melaleuca[C], Thyme[C] **Blends:** Topical Blend[C]

Topical Blend or make blend with equal parts Lavender, Melaleuca and Thyme. 2-3 drops of either blend on area of infection 3x daily for 10 days (dilute with a carrier if there are sensitivities). Follow with Melaleuca for 30 days to assure fungus does not return.

Additional itching relief: Lavender topically

Other oils: Cypress[C], Geranium, Lemongrass, Neroli[C]

Joint conditions

Carpal tunnel	*see* Carpal tunnel
Cartilage injury	*see* Knee injuries
Knee injuries	*see* Knee injuries
Pain	*see* Joint pain
Sprains	*see* Sprains
Stiffness	*see* Arthritis
Tendinitis	*see* Tendinitis
Tennis elbow	*see* Tendinitis
TMJ (temporomandibular joint syndrome)	*see* TMJ

Legend: Preferred, Suggested, Consider

Joint pain
see also Arthritis

Oils: Birch^C, Lemon^{EC}, Lime^C, Peppermint^C, Wintergreen^C **Blends/ Products:** Basic Vitality Supplements^C, Soothing Blend^C, Soothing Blend Rub^C

Apply topically Birch, Soothing Blend (Rub), Lemon, Lime, Peppermint and/or Wintergreen to affected area. Follow with heat pad on low setting. Use carrier oil for sensitive skin. Basic Vitality Supplements used consistently are reported to help.

Other oils: Copaiba^C, Douglas Fir^C, Eucalyptus^{EC}, Ginger^{EC}, Lavender^{EC}, Manuka^C, Marjoram^C, Oregano^{EC}, Siberian Fir^C, Star Anise^C, Turmeric^C

Joy
see Emotional strength

Joyful Blend (elevate your mood)

Blend

Ingredients: Elemi resin, Lavender, Lavandin flower, Lemon Myrtle leaf, Melissa, Osmanthus flower, Sandalwood (Hawaiian), Tangerine peel, Ylang Ylang

Another common formulation: Bergamot, Geranium, Jasmine, Lemon, Mandarin, Palmarosa, Roman Chamomile, Rose, Rosewood, Ylang Ylang

Addresses: Attention deficit, depression, hopelessness, lack of energy, stress

(see Safety Chart, page 23)

Juniper Berry (Juniperus communis)

Properties: Antiseptic, antispasmodic, astringent, disinfectant, diuretic, inflammation, stimulant

Addresses: Arthritis, coughs, dermatitis, diabetes, digestive conditions, eczema, flatulence, kidney stones, UTI, wounds

(see Safety Chart, page 23)

Juvenile diabetes
see Diabetes

Ketones
see Chemical constituents

Kidney failure (renal failure) — see also Kidney stones, UTI

Oils: Clary Sage[C], Lemon, Lemongrass[C] **Blends/Products:** Basic Vitality Supplements, Detoxification Blend/Detoxification Complex[C]

Understand root cause, see infections, cancer and autoimmune diseases. Also consider:

Hydrate with 6-8 glasses of water daily with 1-2 drops Lemon.

Cleanse with Detoxification Complex and Detoxification Blend, plus Basic Vitality Supplements and the Massage Blend Technique.

2-3 drops Clary Sage, Lemongrass and other oils (Massage Blend, Geranium and/or Grapefruit) plus Grounding Blend topically layered over kidney area, follow with warm compress.

Other oils: Geranium, Grapefruit[C] **Blends:** Grounding Blend, Massage Blend,

Kidney infection (pyelonephritis) — see UTI

Kidney stones

Oils: Fennel[EC], Geranium[EC], Lemon[EC], Rosemary **Blends/Products:** Basic Vitality Supplements, Massage Blend

Crisis period:

3-5 8 oz glasses of organic apple juice daily.

5 drops each Geranium, Lemon, Rosemary, 1 Tbsp grade B maple syrup, 2 Tbsp virgin olive oil with 1 cup warm filtered water, mix thoroughly and drink 3x daily until stones dissolve or pass. Also the Massage Blend Technique periodically and 1-2 drops Lemon topically over painful area.

Prevention:

6-8 glasses water with 1-3 drops Lemon daily, Basic Vitality Supplements, avoid caffeine, use filtered water.

Other oils: Eucalyptus[C], Juniper Berry[EC], Roman Chamomile[C]

Legend: Preferred, Suggested, Consider

Kid's Blends *(a collection of blends helpful to children)*

essential oils
Blend

Courage Blend for Children (in a roll-on)

Ingredients: Wild Orange, Amyris Wood, Osmanthus Flower, and Cinnamon Bark in a base of Fractionated Coconut Oil

Addresses: Belief in oneself, confidence, courage, energizing, invigorating , positive mood

Focus Blend for Children (in a roll-on)

Ingredients: Vetiver, Clementine, Peppermint, and Rosemary in a base of Fractionated Coconut Oil

Addresses: Alertness, clarity, enhances focus and learning, uplifting when sad

Grounding Blend for Children (in a roll-on)

Ingredients: Amyris, Balsam Fir, Coriander, and Magnolia in a base of Fractionated Coconut Oil

Addresses: Calming, enhance focus, sooth distress and nervousness

Protective Blend for Children (in a roll-on)

Ingredients: Cedarwood, Litsea, Frankincense, and Rose in a base of Fractionated Coconut Oil

Addresses: Healthy skin, skin irritations, soothing for distress

Restful Blend for Children (in a roll-on)

Ingredients: Lavender, Cananga, Buddha Wood, and Roman Chamomile essential oils in a base of Fractionated Coconut Oil

Addresses: Positive mood, restful atmosphere for sleep, soothing and relaxing

Soothing Blend for Children (in a roll-on)

Ingredients: Copaiba, Lavender, Spearmint, and Zanthoxylum essential oils in a base of Fractionated Coconut Oil

Addresses: Relieves growing pains, relieves tension, sooths muscles for restful sleep, stress-free mood

Safety (for all blends above): Keep out of reach of children under 3. Possible skin sensitivity. If under a doctor's care, consult your physician. Keep out of eyes, inner ears, mouth, and sensitive areas.

Knee injuries   *see also* Sprains

Pain: Birch, White Fir, Wintergreen, Soothing Blend (Rub), Tension Blend

Circulation and warming: Cinnamon Bark, Clove, Cypress, Eucalyptus, Oregano, Peppermint

Encourage tissue repair: Frankincense, Helichrysum, Lemongrass

Use blends of oils recommended to limit pain, increase circulation and encourage tissue repair. Consider Soothing Blend, Cypress, Lemongrass or other combinations. Apply topically to area of discomfort.

Caution: If using Birch, Cypress, Eucalyptus, Lemongrass, Peppermint, White Fir dilute or skin test first. With Cinnamon Bark, Clove, Oregano, Wintergreen definitely dilute with a carrier oil before topical application.

See Sprains for more detailed day-by-day suggestions.

Notes:

Legend: Preferred, Suggested, Consider

L

Labor during pregnancy
see Pregnancy

Lactation
see Breastfeeding

Lactose intolerance
see Food intolerance

Laryngitis

Oils: Frankincense[EC], Lemon[EC] **Blends/Products:** Protective Blend, Protective Blend Throat Drops

Mild: Protective Blend Throat Drops

More help: 2-3 drops Lemon to mouthful water, gargle, swish and swallow. 2-3 drops Frankincense topically to throat.

Serious help: (Submitted by an avid reader of our material.) Add to 15 ml spray bottle with water: 8 drops each Protective Blend, Lemon; 4 drops Peppermint; 2 drops Frankincense and Myrrh; 1 drop Oregano or Thyme, Clove, Sandalwood, Cinnamon Bark. Shake and spray on back of throat. To sweeten add drop of Stevia.

Other oils: Cinnamon Bark, Clove, Geranium[C], Melaleuca[C], Myrrh, Oregano, Peppermint, Rosemary[C], Sandalwood[EC], Thyme[C]

Laundry
see Household care

Lavender *(Lavandula angustifolia)*

essential oil   (also available in a roll-on)

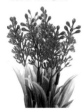

Properties: Analgesic, antibiotic, antidepressant, anti-inflammatory, antiseptic, diuretic, disinfectant, sedative

Addresses: Acne, allergies, arthritic pain, asthma, bronchitis, burns, cold and flu, cuts and wounds, depression, dermatitis, diarrhea, earache, headaches, herpes, hypertension, indigestion, insect bites, insomnia, migraines, muscle pain, nausea, psoriasis, skin disorders, sore throat, stomachache, stress, throat infections

---

Safety charts ... page 23   Special cautions ... page 3   183

Layering

 Definition A procedure of applying 2 or more oils, one after the other, on the same location with 15-60 second interval between.

Leg cramps *see Muscle cramps*

Lemon *(Citrus limon)*

 essential oil

(also available in a roll-on)

Properties: Antibacterial, antibiotic, antiseptic, antiviral, astringent, diuretic

Addresses: Allergies, asthma, cold and flu, constipation, fever, hypertension, insect repellent, sore throat, stomachache, stress, throat infections

(see Safety Chart, page 23)

Lemongrass *(Cymbopogon flexuosus)*

 essential oil

Properties: Analgesic, anti-inflammatory, antiparasitic, antiseptic, astringent, sedative

Addresses: Back pain, constipation, hypertension, indigestion, stomachache, stress

(see Safety Chart, page 23)

Leukemia *see Cancer*

Leukorrhea *see Vaginitis*

Libido, low *(female)* *see also Aphrodisiac*

Oils: Clary Sage^EC, Rose^EC, Ylang Ylang^EC **Blends:** Anti-Aging Blend^C, Blend for Women^C

2-3 drops Clary Sage, Anti-Aging Blend, Blend for Women, Rose or Ylang Ylang bottoms of feet, wrists 2x daily. Also add to a warm bath.

Other oils: Cinnamon Bark^EC, Clove^EC, Geranium^C, Ginger^EC, Jasmine, Peppermint^C, Rosemary^E, Sandalwood^EC, Thyme^E

Legend: Preferred, Suggested, Consider

Libido, low *(male)*   *see also* Aphrodisiac, Erectile dysfunction

Oils: Clary Sage, Sandalwood, Ylang Ylang **Blends:** Basic Vitality Supplements, Joyful Blend

Basic Vitality Supplements consistently plus:

> 2-3 drops Ylang Ylang on reflexology points and 2 drops Clary Sage under tongue daily. (Also Ylang Ylang diluted and applied topically to genital area.)

> Or 3-4 drops each Clary Sage and Ylang Ylang in capsule 1-2x daily.

Other oils: Cinnamon Bark[C], Ginger[C], Jasmine, Myrrh[C], Rosemary

Note: When choosing alternative oils from the list of "**Other oils:**" please review safety precautions on pages 23-28.

Lice

Oils: Eucalyptus[EC], Geranium[EC], Lavender[EC], Lemon[EC], Melaleuca[C]

Depending on severity use one of suggestions below. Identify source, apply to surrounding areas; clothing, bedding, mattress, combs, brushes.

Mild: 2-5 drops Lemon and Melaleuca with 5-10 drops carrier. Mix and apply to scalp, let stand at least 1/2 hour, add 2-5 drops Melaleuca to tsp of shampoo and shampoo. Follow with Melaleuca shampoos daily for week.

Moderate: Use above protocol but double the Melaleuca and after application cover head with shower cap for 1/2 - 1 hour, comb with a lice comb then Melaleuca shampoo. Repeat daily until no signs of lice or nits. Continue Melaleuca shampoos daily for a minimum of 1 week.

Severe: 10 drops Eucalyptus, 5 drops each Geranium, Lavender, Melaleuca with 5-10 drops VCO. Mix and apply to scalp every night, comb with lice comb then cover with shower cap for night. Protect eyes from oils. Next morning Melaleuca shampoo. Repeat complete procedure daily for week.
Other oils: Rosemary[EC] **Blends:** Cleansing Blend, Outdoor Blend[C], Protective Blend

Ligaments   *see* Joint conditions

Lime *(Citrus aurantifolia)*

essential oil

Properties: Antibacterial, antibiotic, antiseptic, disinfectant

Addresses: Cold and flu, fever, hypertension, muscle cramps, respiratory concerns, sore throat, spasms, stress

(see Safety Chart, page 23)

Lip Balm with Essential Oils *(lip moisturizer)* see also Personal care

essential oils
Product

Lip Balms with a natural formula containing plant oils, botanicals, and essential oils to hydrate and soothe lips while delivering the unique scent and taste of essential oils. These extra-moisturizing lip balms contain coconut, moringa seed, and avocado oils along with beeswax to glide easily across the lips, leaving behind hydration that lasts throughout the day.

Three flavors available:
Original: Peppermint and Wild Orange
Tropical: Clementine, Lime and Ylang Ylang
Herbal: Lemon Verbena, Marjoram and Spearmint

Lipoma
see also Tumors

Oils: Frankincense[C], Grapefruit[C] **Blends:** Metabolic Blend, Soothing Blend

1-3 drops each Frankincense and Metabolic Blend (or Grapefruit) topically to area 2x daily. If pain apply Soothing Blend Rub topically.

Other oils: Clove[C], Ginger[C], Sandalwood

Listeria
see Food poisoning

Litsea *(Litsea cubeba)* also known as May Chang

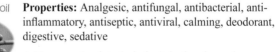

essential oil

Properties: Analgesic, antifungal, antibacterial, anti-inflammatory, antiseptic, antiviral, calming, deodorant, digestive, sedative

Addresses: Anxiety (calming), body odor and excess perspiration, digestive aide, fungal infections, household surface cleaner and disinfectant, insomnia, oily skin,

Legend: Preferred, Suggested, Consider

respiratory stimulant, skin blemishes

(see Safety Chart, page 23)

Liver cancer   *see* Cancer

Liver conditions

Oils: Grapefruit[C], Lemon[E], Myrrh[C] **Blends/Products:** Cellular Complex Blend, Detoxification Blend[C], Detoxification Complex[C], Digestive Enzyme Complex

Identify root cause and consider appropriate protocols. Avoid alcohol and known harmful drugs. Reduce or eliminate sources of toxins such as additives to household and personal care products, insecticides, etc.

Cleanse/strengthen with following with consistency/patience:

Cleanse using Detoxification Complex tablets and 3-5 drops Detoxification Blend topically to liver area daily. (The Detoxification Blend includes Clove, Geranium, Grapefruit and Rosemary, use individually if blend unavailable).

2-5 drops Myrrh topically across back, about bra line, daily.

Basic Vitality Supplements with sufficient hydration, 1-2 drops Lemon per glass of water and periodic Massage Blend Techniques.

Other oils: Clove[C], Geranium[C], Grapefruit[C], Rosemary[EC], Tangerine[C], Turmeric[C] **Blends:** Digestive Blend, Massage Blend

Liver spots   *see* Age spots

Loss of smell   *see* Smell, loss of

Lotions   *see* Personal care and Skin care

essential oils
Product

On occasion applying oils is facilitated by adding the oils to a lotion. Conditions like neuropathy or varicose veins would be examples. There are Hand & Body Lotion products designed and available such that oils can be added directly to the lotion. Other fragrance free lotions can be purchased, made or VCO can be use directly.

Lou Gehrig's disease	*see* ALS

Low blood pressure	*see* Hypotenstion

Lumbago	*see* Back conditions

Lung cancer	*see* Cancer

Lupus	*see also* Autoimmune diseases

Oils: Ginger, Helichrysum[C], Lemon[C], Lemongrass, **Blends/Products:** Basic Vitality Supplements, Detoxification Blend/Detoxification Complex, Digestive Blend, GI Cleansing Formula/Probiotic Defense Formula, Soothing Blend

Nutrition: Basic Vitality Supplements, limit sugars and known food allergies.

Cleanses (*see* Detoxification): GI Cleansing Formula/Probiotic Defense Formula protocol repeated for 3 months. Detoxification Complex with Detoxification Blend for vital organs. Lots of water with 1-3 drops Lemon per glass or 10-12 drops Lemon in a capsule daily.

Inflammation: 4 drops Lemongrass or Helichrysum and Detoxification Blend daily.

Pain: For specific symptoms:

> **Joint pain:** Soothing Blend Rub or Blend topically to area.

> **Digestive discomfort:** Digestive Blend and/or Ginger internally and/or topically.

> **Skin rashes:** Lavender and/or Geranium to soothe.

Further relief: 1 cup Epson Salts with 4 drops each Lavender, Lemongrass, Clove and 2 drops Roman Chamomile. Mix oils with Epson Salts, run hot water bath and dissolve Epson Salts mixture in water and soak for 20 minutes.

Other oils: Clove[EC], Copaiba[C], Frankincense[C], Lavender, Oregano[C] **Blends:** Protective Blend[C]

Legend: Preferred, Suggested, Consider

Lyme disease see also Ticks

Oils: Frankincense[C], Lemongrass, Oregano[C] **Blends/Products:** Basic Vitality Supplements, GI Cleansing Formula/Probiotic Defense Formula, Protective Blend[C]

Lyme disease, as with many other serious health issues, should have treatment that includes professional medical attention.

Antibiotic protocol: 12 drops Protective Blend, 6 drops Oregano, 2 drops Frankincense in capsule. One capsule daily for 14 days, rest 14 days, repeat. During 14 rest days apply 2 drops Lemongrass, 1 drop Oregano on each foot before bedtime. Be aware this is a very strong use of essential oils. Only consider for adults without sensitivities. There can be a possible Herxheimer reaction, if rash or other symptoms reduce daily amounts.

GI Cleansing Formula cleanse: 15 day GI Cleansing Formula/Probiotic Defense Formula procedure, repeat monthly for 3 months, rest 1 month and repeat. (*see* Detoxification)

Supplements: Basic Vitality Supplements, double the omega fatty acids supplement amount, can be taken concurrent with antibiotic protocol and cleanses.

Pain: Consider the Massage Blend Technique periodically.

Three stages of Lyme disease:

Initial infectious stage: Antibiotic protocol above.

If initial phase untreated and later diagnosed: Antibiotic protocol, 14 day rest, GI Cleansing Formula cleanse, repeat sequence if necessary.

Post-Lyme disease syndrome (Infection arrested but symptoms continue): Antibiotics and cleanses may not be necessary but Candida should be considered and address symptoms.

Other oils: Cassia[C], Cinnamon Bark[C], Lavender[C] **Blends:** Cleansing Blend[C], Massage Blend

Lymphatic cancer see Cancer

Lymphatic massage

 De inition A technique to address lymphedema for those who need to do self care. It is best to receive professional training. The basic procedure is:

Lymphatic massage basics: Gentle with very little pressure. No massage oil required, use essential oils. Movements are always towards body trunk but start at trunk and move to extremities. (Confusing? Start close to the trunk of the body and make the short massage motions towards the trunk, then move a little further from the trunk and make the next short motion again toward the trunk, etc, etc.)

Massage motions: Gently press fingers, move skin in circular motion, release. Fingers tight together, gently press, stretch skin by moving fingers apart, twist and release. Gentle sweeping motion toward trunk.

Lymphedema

Oils: Lavender[E], Lime, Peppermint **Blends:** Detoxification Blend, Massage Blend

Mild: 1-3 drops Lavender or Lime topically to area. 1-2 drops Peppermint to bottoms of feet.

Lymphatic self massage:

1-5 drops (depending on area) Massage Blend (or Cypress, Grapefruit, Lavender and Peppermint) with FCO. Gently apply over area. Allow to absorb before massage. One person noted Detoxification Blend added on the lower legs improved results.

See Lymphatic massage and follow procedure.

Manual Lymph Drainage (MLD): Use same oils with a professional massage therapist using MLD.

Other: Consider detoxifying (cleansing) protocols, the Massage Blend Technique periodically and Basic Vitality Supplements.

Other oils: Cypress[C], Grapefruit[C], Helichrysum[C], Lemongrass[C], Rosemary[EC]

Macular degeneration · *see* Eyesight failing

Malaria

Oils: Eucalyptus^{EC}, Melaleuca^C, Oregano^C, Peppermint^{EC}, Thyme^C **Blends/Products:** Detoxification Blend, Detoxification Complex, Repellent Blend^C

Prevention: Take medicines or apply oils that are antiparasitic. Melaleuca, Oregano and Thyme to bottoms of feet or internally. Couple with mosquito repellents; Repellent Blend topically neat and generously to all exposed areas, augment with Eucalyptus and/or Peppermint. Use nets or covering if in the open.

If infected: Cleanse liver with Detoxification Complex and Detoxification Blend protocol. Use antiparasitic oils mentioned above.

Other oils: Basil^E, Cinnamon Bark^E, Clove^C, Lavender^C, Lemon^{EC}, Lemongrass^C **Blends:** Digestive Blend^C

Male hormones · *see* Hormones, male

Manic depression · *see* Bipolar

Magnolia *(Michelia x alba)*

essential oil

Properties: Analgesic, antibacterial, antidepressant, anti-inflammatory, antimicrobial, antiseptic, calming, sedative

Addresses: Anxiety, dry skin, insomnia, irritability, mood swings, nervousness, restlessness, skin blemishes, stress (tension)

(see Safety Chart, page 23)

Manuka

Manuka *(Leptospermum scoparium)*

essential oil

Properties: Analgesic, antibacterial, antidepressant, antifungal, antihistamine, anti-inflammatory, antimicrobial, antiseptic, antiviral, calming, deodorant, decongestant

Addresses: Acne, allergies, bacterial infections, body odor, bronchitis, colds, cuts and scrapes, dandruff, fungal infections, hay fever, insect bites and repellant, joint pain, muscle pain, oily skin, promotes healing of cuts and wounds, rashes, restlessness, skin blemishes, skin lesions and ulcerations, sinus infections, sore throat, strep throat, stress (tension)

(see Safety Chart, page 23)

Marjoram *(Origanum majora)*

essential oil

Properties: Analgesic, antibacterial, antibiotic, antioxidant, antispasmodic, disinfectant, expectorant, sedative

Addresses: Asthma, bronchitis, cold and flu, cough, hypertension, indigestion, insomnia, menstrual problems, migraines, stomachache, stress

(see Safety Chart, page 23)

Massage Blend *(an aromatic blend of oils)*

essential oils
Blend

Ingredients: Basil, Cypress, Grapefruit, Lavender, Marjoram, Peppermint

Another common formulation: Basil, Cypress, Lavender, Marjoram, Peppermint

Addresses: Encourages: relaxation of muscles; reduced stress and tension; increased circulation; soothing of irritated tissue; smoother, improved skin tone

(see Safety Chart, page 23)

Massage Blend Technique

Definition

Stress Management: Lavender, Grounding Blend
Immune support: Melaleuca, Protective Blend
Inflammatory Response: Massage Blend, Soothing Blend

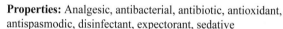

Legend: Preferred, Suggested, Consider

Homeostasis: Peppermint, Wild Orange

A massage like application of 8 essential oils and blends to enhance benefits these oils bring to body and increase feelings of overall health and well-being. See the Helpful Charts section at end of this book for a summary chart of this procedure. This and similar procedures is often taught by essential oils experts.

Mastitis   see Breastfeeding

Mature skin

Age spots (liver spots)	*see* Age spots
Bags under eyes	*see* Bags under eyes
Cellulite reduction	*see* Cellulite reduction
Chapped skin	*see* Chapped skin
Cracked heels	*see* Cracked heels
Dry skin	*see* Chapped skin
Flabby skin	*see* Flabby skin
Skin care	*see* Skin care
Spider veins	*see* Varicose veins
Stretch marks	*see* Stretch marks
Sunspots	*see* Sunspots
Varicose veins	*see* Varicose veins
Wrinkles	*see* Wrinkles

Measles (rubeola)   see also German measles

Oils: Eucalyptus[EC], Lavender[C], Melaleuca[C]

Lavender topically to relieve symptoms of rash. Eucalyptus and Melaleuca internally to minimize the viral infection. Protective Blend as protection if unvaccinated and being in or traveling to an area that may have cases of measles.

Other oils: Coriander **Blends:** Protective Blend

Melaleuca *(Melaleuca alternifolia)*   also known as Tea Tree

essential **◌**oil

used with permission from
© andreas lambriani

(also available in a roll-on)

Properties: Antibacterial, antibiotic, antifungal, anti-inflammatory, antiviral, astringent, disinfectant

Addresses: Acne, cold and flu, cuts and wounds, gum problems, herpes, skin disorders, yeast infection

(see Safety Chart, page 23)

Melanoma   *see* Skin cancer

Melissa *(Melissa officinalis)*

essential **◌**oil

Properties: Analgesic, antidepressant, anti-inflammatory, antiparasitic, antispasmodic, antiviral, digestive, sedative

Addresses: Allergies, anger, anxiety, cold sores, colds, depression, fevers, herpes, hypertension, indigestion, menstrual disorders, migraines, nausea, nervous tension, vertigo, vomiting

Memory   *see also* Mental acuity

[Amnesia]

Oils: Cypress, Frankincense, Geranium, Lemon, Marjoram, Myrrh
Blends: Basic Vitality Supplements, Focus Blend
Long term: Basic Vitality Supplements; 2 drops Frankincense under tongue daily.

Periods of study, etc: diffuse Peppermint or apply Focus Blend.

Immediate: 2-3 drops Focus Blend or Peppermint to temples or inhale.

Any of these oils and blends can be inhaled or applied topically to feet and light massage along spine, to jugular veins or the suboccipital triangle (depression just behind and below the ears).

Other oils: Clary Sage[C], Clove, Lavender, Rosemary[C]

Meniere's disease

Oils: Frankincense, Helichrysum

1-2 drops Frankincense or Helichrysum, apply to back of ear, down jaw line then top of ear and down front to jaw line. Repeat every 1-4 hours.

Consider Candida and use GI Cleansing Formula/Probiotic Defense Formula Candida cleanse.

Other Blends/Products: GI Cleansing Formula/Probiotic Defense Formula

Menopause

see also Emotional conditions, Hormonal balance, Hot flashes, Mood swings, Skin care

General suggestions

Blends/Products: Basic Vitality Supplements, Bone Nutrient Complex, Monthly Blend for Women, Phytoestrogen Complex

Consistent Basic Vitality Supplements and Phytoestrogen Complex (perimenopausal 1-2 capsules daily with food, post-menopausal 2 capsules daily with food). 1-2 drops Monthly Blend for Women bottoms of feet, back of neck, temples or inhale. 4 capsules Bone Nutrient Complex daily.

Reduce stress

Oils: Bergamot[C], Frankincense[C], Roman Chamomile[C], Sandalwood[C]
Blends: Massage Blend

2-3 drops Sandalwood or 1 drop each Bergamot, Frankincense and Roman Chamomile mixed together. Apply to the bottoms of the feet, the back of the neck, the temples and/or inhale the aroma.

The Massage Blend Technique twice a month at least, more often if needed.

Increase natural progesterone

Oils: Frankincense[C], Geranium[C], Oregano[C], Thyme[C]

Use natural sources (many identified online), Basic Vitality Supplements, 1-2 drops Thyme and/or Oregano to bottoms of feet (limit Oregano to 8-10 days in succession). Geranium topically over liver, adrenal glands and/or kidneys.

Help symptoms

Fatigue: Ginger, Peppermint, White Fir, Basic Vitality Supplements, Energy & Stamina Complex

Peppermint and White Fir inhaled or on temples, Ginger topically to liver and adrenal glands. Basic Vitality Supplements and Energy & Stamina Complex.

Hot flashes: Citrus oils, Clary Sage[C], Geranium[C], Grounding Blend[C], Monthly Blend for Women[C], Peppermint[C]

Peppermint on feet at night, back of neck, chest or spray bottle with Peppermint and water. Others prefer or use Monthly Blend for Women additionally on ankles or other oils above.

Insomnia: Restful Blend[C], Lavender, Roman Chamomile[C], Sandalwood[C]

Inhale or on pillow at night.

Libido: Clary Sage[C], Ginger, Joyful Blend[C], Peppermint, Ylang Ylang[C]

Diffuse or use as perfume.

Memory loss: Frankincense, Peppermint, Rosemary

Diffuse or apply to temples and back of neck.

Other oils: Basil[C], Cardamom[C], Clary Sage[C], Cypress[EC], Fennel[E], Geranium[C], Lavender[C], Peppermint, Roman Chamomile[EC], Thyme[C], Wild Orange[C], Ylang Ylang **Blends:** Grounding Blend[C], Restful Blend[C]

Menorrhagia *(heavy, prolonged menstrual periods)*
see also Hormonal balance

Oils: Clary Sage, Cypress[EC], Rose[EC] **Blends/Products:** Basic Vitality Supplements, Cellular Complex Blend, Monthly Blend for Women, Phytoestrogen Complex

Phytoestrogen Complex and Monthly Blend for Women are specifically formulated to balance hormones and manage menstrual problems.

Also found helpful is consistent Basic Vitality Supplements, 8 drops or 1 capsule Cellular Complex Blend and 2-3 drops Frankincense under tongue daily.

Also Clary Sage, Cypress and Metabolic Blend topically applied to lower abdomen. For additional help use warm compress after applying oils and cup and inhale. (Note: Leading eo experts and many others point out that different oils work for different folks and there is usually a need to do some experimentation to determine what works best for each individual.)

Other oils: Geranium[C], Roman Chamomile[C] **Blends/Products:** Metabolic Blend

Menstrual conditions *see also* Hormonal balance

Amenorrhoea (absence of)	*see* Amenorrhoea
Dysmenorrhoea (cramps, painful)	*see* Dysmenorrhoea
Endometriosis	*see* Endometriosis
Menorrhagia (heavy, prolonged)	*see* Menorrhagia
Oligomenorrhea (irregular, scanty)	*see* Oligomenorrhea
PCOS (polycystic ovary syndrome)	*see* PCOS
Uterine fibroids	*see* Uterine fibroids

Mental acuity *(alertness, concentration, cognitive impairment)*

see also Memory

Oils: Frankincense[C], Peppermint[EC], Vetiver[C] **Blends:** Basic Vitality Supplements, Focus Blend, Grounding Blend[C], Joyful Blend[C]

Long term: Basic Vitality Supplements; 2 drops Frankincense under tongue daily.

Alertness: 2-3 drops Joyful Blend, Focus Blend or Peppermint to temples or inhale.

Concentration: Grounding Blend, Focus Blend or Vetiver, inhale or bottoms of feet.

Any of these oils and blends can be inhaled or applied topically to feet, with light massage along spine, to jugular veins or the suboccipital triangle (depression just behind and below the ears).

Other oils: Basil[EC], Cardamom[EC], Invigorating Blend[C], Lavender[C], Lemon[C], Melissa[C], Patchouli[C], Petitgrain[C], Rosemary[EC]

Mental conditions

see also Emotional conditions or Personality disorders

Alzheimer's	*see* Alzheimer's
Bipolar (manic depression)	*see* Bipolar
Confusion	*see* Mental acuity
Dementia	*see* Dementia
Depression	*see* Depression
Fatigue	*see* Mental acuity
Memory loss (amnesia)	*see* Memory
Mental acuity	*see* Mental acuity
OCD (obsessive compulsive disorder)	*see* OCD
Paranoia	*see* Paranoia
Postpartum depression	*see* Pregnancy
PTSD (post traumatic stress disorder)	*see* Stress
Schizophrenia	*see* Schizophrenia
Stress (strain)	*see* Stress

Metabolic Blend *(a slimming help)*

Blend

(also available in Sofgels)

Ingredients: Cinnamon Bark, Ginger, Grapefruit, Lemon, Peppermint

Addresses: Appetite, calms stomach, hunger management, lifts mood, proper hydration

(see Safety Chart, page 23)

Metabolic Blend products

Product

Complementary products to the Metabolic Blend for weight management include:

Softgel: Metabolic blend in an easy and convenient softgel.

Trim shakes: Chocolate, Orange Cream, Vanilla and Vegetarian shakes that are convenient and delicious shake mixes providing essential nutrients of a healthy meal with only 125 calories per serving that can replace one meal per day.

Gum: Sugar free gum provides one drop of Meatabolic Blend

Legend: Preferred, Suggested, Consider

conveniently to help reduce appetite and manage portions sizes.

Basic Vitality Supplements: These healthy additions are also recommended. *see* Basic Vitality Supplements

(see Safety Chart, page 23)

Metabolic syndrome

Oils: Coriander[C], Cypress[CE], Helichrysum[C], Lavender[EC], Lemongrass[C], Marjoram **Blends/Products:** Basic Vitality Supplements, Grounding Blend[C], Yarrow-Pomegranate Blend

Basic Vitality Supplements are a must.

Heart problems: Equal parts Cypress, Helichrysum, Lavender and Marjoram topically to the chest area over heart, bottoms of feet and the wrists at least 2x daily.

Diabetes: Grounding Blend on feet in morning, 8-10 drops Coriander in capsule daily, Lavender on feet at night.

Cholesterol: 5-6 drops Lemongrass in capsule daily, adequate levels of water daily.

Other oils: Basil[C], Cassia[C], Ylang Ylang[EC] **Blends:** Protective Blend[C]

Migraine headache   *see also* Headache

Oils: Frankincense **Blends:** Soothing Blend[C], Tension Blend[C]

Migraines are very individual and successful oils will also vary. Listed here are two protocols that worked for others, experiment.

Experience 1: Start at first warning signs. 1-2 drops Frankincense from thumb to roof of mouth. Roll Tension Blend on back of neck and base of skull. 1-2 drops Soothing Blend on temples and forehead. 1-2 drops Digestive Blend internally if nauseated. Repeat every 15 minutes - 2 hours as long as necessary. Nap if possible.

Experience 2: Start as soon as warning appears. 1-2 drops Tension Blend on forehead continue over crown of head through hair to neck and shoulders, rub into each area. Repeat every 15 minutes - 2 hours as long as necessary. Nap if able.

Other oils: Basil[EC], Copaiba[C], Cumin[C], Eucalyptus[EC], Lavender[E], Marjoram[E], Peppermint[EC], Spikenard[C]

Mildew
see Mold and Mildew

Miscarriage
see Pregnancy

Mites
see Allergies, Insect repellent, Scabies

Moisturizing
see Personal care and Skin care

Mold allergy
see Allergies

Mold and mildew
see also Household cleaning

Oils: Lemon **Blends:** Cleansing Blend[C], Protective Blend[C]

Antifungal oils: Cinnamon Bark[C], Clove[C], Geranium[E], Melaleuca[E], Oregano[C], Rosemary[C], Thyme[C]

Surfaces: 8-10 drops Protective Blend in 8 oz spray bottle with water. Augment with any antifungal oils. To improve odor add Lemon or Peppermint.

Fruits and vegetables: 5-10 drops Lemon or Protective Blend in sink of water, place produce in colander and agitate in sink, dry.

Fabrics: 3-4 drops Protective Blend to wash cycle, 1-2 drops Cleansing Blend on wash cloth, add to dryer.

Airborne: Protective Blend or Cleansing Blend on an air filter (AC/heater or purifier in home. Diffuse any of antifungal oils.

Other oils: Lavender, Peppermint **Blends:** Invigorating Blend

Moles

Oils: Frankincense

Apply 1 drop Frankincense topically directly to mole 2x daily. Can take 4 - 6 weeks before falling off.

Some suggest Oregano. This is a "hot" oil, apply only on mole and not surrounding area, use caution.

Caution: If mole is changing in shape, size or color seek professional help.

Molluscum warts   *see* Warts

Mononucleosis *(infectious mononucleosis)*

Oils: Frankincense^C, Oregano^C **Blends:** Protective Blend^C

Make capsules with 6 drops Protective Blend, 3 drops Oregano and 2 drops Frankincense, take 3x daily with meals until symptoms subside; 2x daily for 2 more days. Be aware this is a strong use of essential oils. Only consider for adults without sensitivities. There can be a possible Herxheimer reaction, if rash or other symptoms reduce daily amounts.

Additional help/protection: Diffuse Respiratory Blend and take Basic Vitality Supplements.

Other oils: Lemon^C **Blends:** Respiratory Blend^C, GI Cleansing Formula/ Probiotic Defense Formula, Basic Vitality Supplements

Monoterpenes   *see* Chemical constituents

Montezuma's revenge   *see* Diarrhea

Monthly Blend for Women *(gives clarity and calm)*

(comes in roll-on)

essential oils
Blend

Ingredients: Bergamot, Carrot Seed, Cedarwood, Clary Sage, Fennel, Geranium, Lavender, Palmarosa herb, Roman Chamomile, Vitex plant, Ylang Ylang

Another common formulation: Clary Sage, Fennel, Jasmine, Lavender, Marjoram, Yarrow

Addresses: Cramps, emotional swings, hot flashes, nausea

(see Safety Chart, page 23)

Mood swings

see also Bipolar, Depression, Emotional conditions, Hormonal balance, PMS

Oils: Frankincense^C, Lavender^C, Rosemary^C **Blends/Products:** Basic Vitality Supplements, Grounding Blend^C, Invigorating Blend, Joyful Blend^C, Monthly Blend for Women, Restful Blend^C

Basic Vitality Supplements with 2 drops Frankincense under tongue daily.

From the following oils diffuse and/or apply topically behind ears, on wrists or bottoms of feet 2-3x daily.

Hormonal: Monthly Blend for Women, Blend for Women
Other: Choose blend based on mood needs.
Grounding Blend: Grounding, Reassuring, Consoling
Invigorating Blend: Invigorating, Stimulating, Motivating
Joyful Blend: Inspiring, Encouraging, Cheering
Restful Blend: Calming, Composing, Placating
Self made blend: 6d Geranium, 2d Clary Sage, 3d Ylang Ylang

Other oils: Blue Tansy[C], Clary Sage[C], Geranium[C], Jasmine[C], Magnolia[C], Neroli[EC], Peppermint[C], Roman Chamomile[C], Rose[C], Spearmint[C], Tangerine[C], Wild Orange[C], Ylang Ylang[C] **Blends/Products:** Blend for Women, Phytoestrogen Complex

Morning sickness
see Pregnancy

Moroccan Chamomile
see Blue Tansy

Mosquito bites
see also Insect repellent, Skeeter syndrome

Oils: Lavender[C] **Blends:** Outdoor Blend[C]
Dab oil topically, directly on area bitten as soon as possible. Repeat if necessary every 1 to 2 hours. For young children or very sensitive skin dilute oils with a carrier.

Other oils: Lemongrass, Melaleuca

Moths
see Insect repellent

Motion sickness (car sick, sea sick)

Oils: Coriander[C], Peppermint[EC] **Blends:** Digestive Blend[C]

Before travel: Inhale Digestive Blend or other oil using an inhaler or cup & inhale. Some find it effective to rub 1-2 drops of Coriander or other oils behind ears.

Legend: Preferred, Suggested, Consider

After upset: 3-5 drops internally with water, juice or in capsule. Or rub on abdomen or for children on tummy with carrier oil.

Other oils: Fennel^E, Ginger^{EC}

Motivation   *see* Emotional strength

Mouth, inflammation of the   *see* Stomatitis

MRSA   *see also* Staph infection

Oils: Frankincense^C, Oregano^C **Blends:** Protective Blend^C

4 drops each Protective Blend and Oregano in capsule 2-3x daily for 2 weeks. Or 4 drops each of Oregano and Melaleuca, 1 drop Frankincense in capsule 2-3x daily. Diffuse with 2 drops each Protective Blend and Oregano.

Open sores: Apply topically Frankincense or layer Anti-Aging Blend, Protective Blend, Oregano and Frankincense. Apply cautiously to avoid cross- contamination to other areas or other people. A carrier may be used. Consider Protective Blend with carrier around the wound.

Additional protection: Use the Massage Blend Technique periodically.

Other oils: Cinnamon Bark^C, Clove^C, Dill^C, Eucalyptus^C, Lemongrass^C, Lemon^C, Melaleuca^C, Thyme^C **Blends:** Anti-Aging Blend, Massage Blend

Note: When choosing alternative oils from the list of "**Other oils:**" please review safety precautions on pages 23-28.

Mucolytic   *see* Congestion

Multiple sclerosis   *see also* Autoimmune diseases

Oils: Frankincense^C, Lemon^C, Peppermint^C **Blends/Products:** Basic Vitality Supplements, Invigorating Blend, Protective Blend

Daily to reduce symptoms: Basic Vitality Supplements, mornings Peppermint to bottoms of feet, during day 1-3 drops Lemon to each glass water (drink lots), evening Frankincense to bottoms of feet.

Flare up: Layer Peppermint and Frankincense on bottoms of feet and/or affected area.

Choking: 2-3 drops Frankincense in shot glass half full of water aand sip slowly between coughs.

Discouraged: Diffuse Invigorating Blend or other uplifting oils.

Prevent infectious disease: Diffuse Protective Blend or Cleansing Blend regularly.

Also consider: Helichrysum (supports nerve tissue regeneration), Sandalwood (antibacterial, antiviral, soothing), Clove (strong anti-pathogenic properties).

Other oils: Clove, Helichrysum, Melaleuca[C], Sandalwood[C] **Blends:** Cleansing Blend

Muscle cramps *(muscle spasms)*   *see also* Nerve damage

Oils: Cypress[C], Marjoram[C], Petitgrain[EC] **Blends/Products:** Basic Vitality Supplements, Soothing Blend[C]

Immediate relief: 2-5 drops Massage Blend, Soothing Blend or Tension Blend directly to muscle area affected with massage strokes.

Spasms: Muscular or nervous spasms (involuntary contractions) are said to be relieved with topical or internal use of Petitgrain.

Long term: Basic Vitality Supplements. Periodic Massage Blend Technique.

Other oils: Basil[C], Bergamot[C], Blue Tansy, Frankincense[C], Lime[C], Peppermint[C], Ravensara, Roman Chamomile[EC], Star Anise[C] **Blends:** Massage Blend, Tension Blend

Muscle pain *(muscle stiffness)*

Oils: Birch[C], Lavender[C], Marjoram, Peppermint[C] **Blends/Products:** Basic Vitality Supplements, Soothing Blend[C]

Apply oils topically to affected area (dilute with FCO for larger areas and sensitive skin).

Pain relief: Birch, Lavender or Soothing Blend

Calm, relax and improve circulation: Massage Blend, Lavender, Marjoram and/or Rosemary

Legend: Preferred, Suggested, Consider

Other oils: Basil, Blue Tansy, Copaiba^C, Douglas Fir^C, Lemongrass, Manuka^C, Oregano^{EC}, Ravensara, Rosemary^{EC}, Siberian Fir^C, Thyme^{EC}, Turmeric^C, White Fir^C, Wintergreen^C **Blends:** Massage Blend^C, Tension Blend

Muscle testing

Muscle testing is a technique to identify what and how much of an oil or other remedy might be effective.

An example of an American Indian way: Hold the product to your chest. Pause with the thought that your body will tell you if the product is good for you. If you fall or slightly float forward, your body is vibrating that you need the product. If you fall backwards, you should not take the product.

Muscular dystrophy

Oils: Frankincense, Lemon^C, Lemongrass^C, Marjoram^C **Blends/Products:** Basic Vitality Supplements, Massage Blend^C, Soothing Blend^C

Basic nutrition: Basic Vitality Supplements, foods high in antioxidants, fruits, raw vegetables, good meats. Avoid carbohydrates, processed foods, trans-fats, alcohol, caffeine, carbonated drinks. Drink sufficient water daily with 1-3 drops Lemon.

2 drops Frankincense under tongue daily and 1-2 Massage Blend Techniques each week.

Muscle discomfort: Soothing Blend, Lemongrass and Marjoram.

Because of the variety of types and progression try and experiment with other oils for specific symptoms and conditions.

Other oils: Basil^C, Eucalyptus^C, Lavender^C, Geranium^C, Ginger^C, Rosemary^C

Myocardial infarction
see Heart conditions

Myrrh *(Commiphora myrrha)*

essential oil

Properties: Analgesic, antibacterial, antibiotic, antifungal, anti-inflammatory, antiseptic, astringent, decongestant, expectorant, sedative

Addresses: Cough, cuts and wounds, dermatitis, diarrhea, gum/mouth problems, hemorrhoids, indigestion, skin disorders, stomachache, yeast infection

(see Safety Chart, page 23)

Notes:

Legend: Preferred, Suggested, Consider

Nail fungus

[finger, toe]

Oils: Melaleuca, Oregano^C **Blends/Products:** GI Cleansing Formula/ Probiotic Defense Formula, Topical Blend^C

Some require stronger protocols, usually takes 3-10 weeks, normally nail will turn yellow or black during the process. Replace emery boards and sterilize other manicure/pedicure tools.

Mild: 2-3 drops Topical Blend, Melaleuca or Oregano directly to nail 2-4 times daily, continue 2 weeks after.

Moderate: Above plus GI Cleansing Formula, 3 capsules daily with meals for 10 days, follow with Probiotic Defense Formula, 3 capsules daily with meals for 5 days, rest 10 days, repeat 2x if necessary.

Strong: Some have found they need to couple above protocols with a serious diet eliminating yeast and acidic foods.

Other oils: Clove, Frankincense, Geranium, Lemon, Lemongrass, Neroli^C, Rosemary

Nails, strengthen

Oils: Lemon^EC **Blends/Products:** Basic Vitality Supplements

Basic Vitality Supplements consistently and/or topical application of 1 drop Lemon daily.

If abnormalities continue consider possibility of other health concerns.

Other oils: Frankincense^C, Grapefruit^C, Myrrh^C **Blends:** Invigorating Blend^C

Narcolepsy   *see also* Autoimmune diseases

Oils: Peppermint **Blends/Products:** Basic Vitality Supplements, Grounding Blend, Joyful Blend, Restful Blend, Energy & Stamina Complex

Long term: Nutrition with Basic Vitality Supplements and wholesome eating habits. Regular sleep patterns helped with Grounding Blend, Joyful Blend and Restful Blend.

Immediate helps: Inhale Peppermint or apply topically to forehead, temples or back of neck. Diffuse Peppermint or Wild Orange. Use Energy & Stamina Complex rather than harmful stimulants.

Other oils: Lavender, Wild Orange **Blends:** Focus Blend, Invigorating Blend

Nasal congestion
see Congestion

Nasal irrigation
see Neti pot

Nausea

Oils: Cardamom^{EC}, Coriander^C **Blends:** Digestive Blend^C

1-5 drops Digestive Blend or other oils mentioned. Inhale from bottle or with inhaler. Internally with water, juice or capsule. Topically on abdomen with carrier for children, on bottoms of feet for small infants. Repeat as soon as 10-15 minutes if necessary for relief.

Other oils: Fennel^E, Ginger^{EC}, Peppermint^{EC}, Spikenard^C, Yarrow^C

Neat

 Definition A common term used to describe using essential oils topically without diluting them with a carrier oil. Just applying them directly without dilution.

Neck pain
see Back conditions

Neroli *(Citrus aurantium)*

essential oil (comes in roll-on)

Properties: Antibacterial, antidepressant, anti-infectious, antiparasitic, antiseptic, antispasmodic, antiviral, aphrodisiac, astringent, calming, deodorant, digestive, sedative

Addresses: Anxiety (fear), aphrodisiac, arrhythmia, chronic diarrhea, colic, depression, fibrillation, hysteria, insomnia,

Legend: Preferred, Suggested, Consider

nervous indigestion, nervousness, palpitations, PMS, sensitive skin, shock, skin care (chapped skin, dry skin, itchy skin, mature skin, wrinkles), stress (tension), stretch marks

(see Safety Chart, page 23)

Nerve conditions

Bell's Palsy	*see* Bell's Palsy
Facial neuralgia	*see* Neuralgia
Nerve damage	*see* Nerve damage
Neuralgia	*see* Neuralgia
Neuropathy	*see* Neuropathy
Trigeminal neuralgia	*see* Neuralgia

Nerve damage

Oils: Frankincense, Helichrysum

Help nerve tissue restoration: 1-2 drops Helichrysum topically to area of injury 2-3x daily.

Help nerve tissue and increase circulation: 3-4 drops of this blend to area of injury 2-3x daily. 5 parts Helichrysum, 3 parts Cypress, 8 parts Geranium, 1 part Peppermint.

Pain: Use Soothing Blend also if pain management required.

Other oils: Cypress, Geranium, Peppermint, Roman Chamomile **Blends:** Grounding Blend, Massage Blend, Soothing Blend

Nervous exhaustion   see Fatigue, emotional

Nervous vomiting   see Vomiting

Nervousness   see Anxiety

Neti pot

Definition A device that allows one to flush the nasal passages and sinus area with a mixture of water and essential oils. Neti pots are available at most drug stores. A new version of sinus irrigator is battery operated and easier to use.

Neuralgia

[trigeminal neuralgia]

Oils: Eucalyptus[EC], Frankincense[C], Helichrysum[E]

1-2 drops Frankincense on pain points, crown of head and under tongue 2x daily. Also base of skull.

Other oils: Lavender[C], Marjoram[C], Roman Chamomile[EC] **Blends:** Soothing Blend

Neuropathy

Oils: Basil[C], Cypress[C], Marjoram[C], Peppermint **Blends:** Massage Blend[C]

Protocol 1: Add 20-30 drops each Massage Blend and Cypress to 6-8 oz of lotion (Hand & Body Lotion or VCO) and apply topically to area 2x daily. Cover with hot moist towel, plastic bag and dry towel after application. *see also* Lotions.

Protocol 2: Rub 2-4 drops each Basil, Cypress and Marjoram into foot; finish with 2-4 drops Peppermint then cover with hot moist towel, plastic bag and dry towel. Repeat on other foot.

Other oils: Coriander[C], Eucalyptus[C], Grapefruit[C], Lavender[C], Lemongrass[C], Wintergreen[C] **Blends:** Grounding Blend

Nose/throat conditions

Congestion	*see* Congestion
Nosebleed	*see* Nosebleed
Laryngitis	*see* Laryngitis
Polyp, nasal	*see* Polyp
Smell, loss of	*see* Smell (loss of)
Sore throat	*see* Sore throat
Strep throat	*see* Sore throat
Stuffy nose	*see* Allergies or Colds
Tonsillitis	*see* Tonsillitis

Legend: Preferred, Suggested, Consider

Nosebleed (bloody nose)

Oils: Frankincense[EC], Helichrysum[C]

2-3 drops Helichrysum to nostril either external or internal using a Q-tip or tissue saturated with oil.

Other oils: Cypress[EC], Lavender[C], Lemon[EC]

Nursing
see Breastfeeding

Nurturing
see Emotional strength

Nutritional supplements
see Basic Vitality Supplements

Nuts allergy
see Allergies

Obesity
see Weight loss

Obsessive compulsive disorder (OCD)

Oils: Patchouli **Blends:** Grounding Blend

1-2 drops Patchouli or Grounding Blend in roller bottle, apply behind ears, on wrists, bottoms of feet and/or along spine 2-3x daily. Also diffuse or cup & inhale.

Other oils: Cypress[C], Frankincense, Geranium[C], Lavender[C], Ylang Ylang[C]

OCD
see Obsessive compulsive disorder

Odynophagia
see Swallowing difficulty

Oil pulling

Definition This is a procedure used to support oral health and help minimize pathogens overall. Some even suggest it helps to prevent disease.

Prior to breakfast, on an empty stomach, add 3-6 drops essential oil to 1 Tbsp FCO or other carrier. Take mixture into mouth but do not swallow. Hold and move mixture slowly in mouth as if rinsing or swishing, "suck and pull through the teeth" for up to 15-20 minutes (even 2 minutes is helpful). When finished, spit from the mouth, do not swallow. Thoroughly rinse and wash mouth; brush with Protective Blend toothpaste.

Oily skin

Oils: Lemon[C] **Blends/Products:** Topical Blend Foaming Face Wash

Cleanse with Topical Blend Foaming Face Wash or with 1 oz Coconut Oil and 12-30 drops Lemon.

Other products: Essential oils based Facial Cleanser *(see* Skin care), Litsea[C], Manuka[C]

Ointment, skin   *see* Essential Ointment

Oligomenorrhea *(irregular or scanty menstrual periods)*
see also Hormonal balance

Oils: Clary Sage[EC], Fennel[EC], Peppermint[EC], Rosemary[EC] **Blends:** Monthly Blend for Women, Phytoestrogen Complex

Phytoestrogen Complex and Monthly Blend for Women are specifically formulated to balance hormones and manage menstrual problems.

> **Phytoestrogen Complex:** For pre-menopausal women it is suggested 1-2 capsules daily with food or as needed.

> **Monthly Blend for Women:** Available in a roller bottle for topical application to back of the neck, temples and bottoms of feet.

Also consider using other oils recommended. (Leading essential oils experts and many others point out that different oils work for different folks and there is usually a need to do some experimentation to determine what works best for each individual.)

Note: Fennel seems to be recommended more often than others. For additional help cup & inhale and/or apply oils topically to lower abdomen and use a warm compress following application.

Other oils: Lavender[EC], Melissa[EC], Rose[EC], Yarrow[C]

Omega-3 Fish Oil

 Product Omega-3 fish oil supplements are important nutritional supplements available in easy to swallow and great tasting liquid form. Some provide 1,000 mg of pure fish oil per serving. Omega-3 fish oil contains essential nutrients EPA and DHA to support healthy brain, cardiovascular, immune and joint function. There are products available with no fishy taste which are great for children and others that are unable to take capsules.

Open sores
see Ulcerations, skin

Oral hygiene
see also Bad breath

Oils: Myrrh[EC] **Blends/Products:** Protective Blend[C], Protective Blend Toothpaste

Regular teeth care: 2x daily floss and brush with Protective Blend Toothpaste or directly with 3-4 drops Protective Blend.

Gum health: 1-4 drops Protective Blend in 1 Tbsp water or carrier oil. Swish and pull mixture through teeth for 5-10 minutes 2x daily, do not swallow. Add Lemon or Peppermint to improve taste. Strengthen by adding 1-2 drops Myrhh.

Other oils: Green Mandarin[C], Lemon[C], Melaleuca[C], Peppermint

Orange
see Wild Orange

Oregano *(Origanum vulgare)*

(also available in a roll-on)

Properties: Antibacterial, antibiotic, antiparasitic, antiviral, disinfectant

Addresses: Cold and flu, diarrhea, immune strengthener, sore throat, throat infection, yeast infection

(see Safety Chart, page 23)

Osteoarthritis
see Arthritis

Osteomyelitis
see also MRSA

Oils: Frankincense, Helichrysum, Peppermint **Blends:** Protective Blend

One combination suggested is to topically apply to area 2-3 drops each Protective Blend, Frankincense, Helichrysum and Peppermint. Layer them (apply individually 30-60 sec apart). Also take your choice of above oils in capsule, 4 drops each. Repeat 2-3x daily. May take weeks.

Also consider Probiotic Defense Formula and Basic Vitality Supplements.

Other oils: Eucalyptus, Melaleuca

Osteoporosis

Oils: Cypress, Helichrysum, Oregano **Blends/Products:** Basic Vitality Supplements, Bone Nutrient Complex, Grounding Blend, Phytoestrogen Complex^C, Soothing Blend^C

Foundation: Basic Vitality Supplements, Phytoestrogen Complex with Bone Nutrient Complex and consistent, regular weight-bearing exercise.

Pain: Apply Soothing Blend Rub.

Strengthen bones: Apply 2-5 drops Soothing Blend and Cypress before retiring and Helichrysum upon arising. Also consider Oregano (a "hot" oil, may require dilution) and Grounding Blend.

Other oils: Eucalyptus, Frankincense, Geranium^C, Lemon^C, Rosemary^C, Wintergreen^C

Outdoor Blend *(shield against insects)*

Blend

Ingredients: Arborvitae, Catnip, Cedarwood, Lemon Eucalyptus, Litsea, Nootka, Vanilla Bean Absolute, Ylang Ylang and with Tamanu oil that provides added support.

Addresses: Protection from and reducing effects of insect bites and stings.

Spray: Available in handy spray bottle.

(see Safety Chart, page 23)

Ovarian cancer
see Cancer

Legend: Preferred, Suggested, Consider

Ovarian cyst
see also Cysts

Oils: Frankincense[C], Sandalwood

Soak end of organic tampon in 8-10 drops Frankincense and Sandalwood with 1 tsp carrier oil, insert at night before retiring. Repeat nightly.

Other oils: Basil[C], Clary Sage, Cypress, Geranium, Lavender, Myrrh

Overeating
see Obesity

Overweight
see Weight loss

Oxides
see Chemical constituents

Oxygenated compounds
see Chemical constituents

Notes:

Legend: Preferred, Suggested, Consider

PAD   *see* Heart conditions

Pain *(analgesic)*   *see also* Headache and Muscle Pain

[Chronic pain]

Oils: Peppermint[EC] **Blends:** Massage Blend, Soothing Blend[C] (Blend, Capsule, Rub), Tension Blend

Muscle and Joint: Soothing Blend and Soothing Blend Rub. Massage Blend is more soothing for some types of pain. *see* Muscle pain.

Chronic: The Massage Blend Technique periodically.

Headache: Peppermint, Tension Blend. *see* Headache.

Other combinations of the oils listed below have proven effective for others. Experiment to find your best combination. This is a partial list of oils with analgesic properties:

Oils: Birch[C], Blue Tansy[C], Cypress[C], Eucalyptus[EC], Lavender[EC], Lemongrass[C], Marjoram[EC], Melaleuca[C], Peppermint[EC], White Fir[C], Wintergreen[EC], Black Pepper[C], Cedarwood, Copaiba[C], Douglas Fir[C], Elemi[C], Frankincense[C], Ginger[C], Grapefruit[C], Helichrysum[C], Lemon[C], Lime, Myrrh[C], Siberian Fir[C], Spearmint[C], Tangerine[C], Vetiver, Wild Orange[C], Ylang Ylang[C], Bergamot[C], Cilantro[C], Clove[C], Coroiander[C], Geranium[EC], Jasmine[C], Oregano[C], Ravensara[C], Roman Chamomile[E], Rosemary[EC]

Painting   *see* Household care

Palpitations   *see* Heart conditions

Pancreatitis

Oils: Cypress[C], Fennel[C], Lemon[EC] **Blends:** Digestive Blend, Protective Blend[C]

Pain: 2-3 drops Digestive Blend topically to abdomen and/or Lemon and Marjoram to pancreas area and reflexology points on feet.

Infection: Protective Blend internally and on bottoms of feet.

On going support: GI Cleansing Formula/Probiotic Defense Formula cleanse, Basic Vitality Supplements. 1-3 drops Lemon each glass of water. Also consider Cellular Complex Blend, Fennel and Cypress to pancreas and reflexology points on feet.

Other oils: Basil[C], Coriander[C], Cinnamon Bark[C], Geranium[C], Helichrysum[C], Marjoram, Rosemary[C] **Blends:** Cellular Complex Blend, GI Cleansing Formula/Probiotic Defense Formula

Panic attack   *see* Anxiety

Paralysis   *see also* Stroke

Oils: Frankincense, Helichrysum[C], Peppermint[EC] **Blends:** Grounding Blend, Massage Blend

Serious conditions require professional medical help. Experiences suggest oils helpful for temporary conditions and can be comforting for more serious conditions.

Soothing/revitalizing: The Massage Blend Technique periodically and/or Grounding Blend.

Stimulating: Peppermint.

Helpful for tissue: Apply 1-5 drops Helichrysum and Frankincense to spine, crown of head and bottoms of feet.

Other oils: Basil[EC], Cypress[C], Geranium[C], Ginger[C], Lavender[E], Lemongrass[C] **Blends:/Products** Cleansing Blend[C], Respiratory Blend[C]

Paranoia

Blends/Products: Basic Vitality Supplements, Grounding Blend, Joyful Blend, Restful Blend

1-2 drops Grounding Blend, Joyful Blend or Restful Blend in roller bottle, apply behind ears, on wrists, bottoms of feet and/or along spine 2-3x daily. Also diffuse or cup & inhale. Basic Vitality Supplements for nutritional foundation.

Some suggest cleansing gut with GI Cleansing Formula/Probiotic Defense Formula and/or cleansing the liver with Detoxification Blend, Detoxification Complex.

Other oils: Frankincense, White Fir **Blends/Products:** Detoxification Blend^C, Detoxification Complex^C, GI Cleansing Formula/Probiotic Defense Formula

Parasite infections

Intestinal parasites
see also Antiparasitic, Amoebic dysentery, Diarrhea
[Protozoa, Round worms, Tapeworms, Flukes]

Oils: Lavender^C, Lemon^EC, Melaleuca^C, Oregano^C **Blends:** Digestive Blend^C, GI Cleansing Formula, Protective Blend

Strong: 3-4 drops each Protective Blend, Oregano, Lemon and Melaleuca in capsule, 2x daily.

Mild: 3-4 drops Lavender in a capsule 2-3x daily.

Also effective: GI Cleansing Formula capsule 2-4x daily plus Digestive Blend internally or topically to stomach.

Other oils: Arborvitae^C, Cinnamon Bark^E, Roman Chamomile^EC, Tangerine^C , Thyme^EC **Blends:** Cleansing Blend

Note: When choosing alternative oils from the list of "**Other oils:**" please review safety precautions on pages 23-28.

Skin Parasites
see also Antiparasitic, Lice, Scabies

Oils: Lavender^EC, Melaleuca^C **Blends:** Cellular Complex Blend^C, Outdoor Blend^C, Protective Blend^C, Topical Blend^C

Cellular Complex Blend topically to area plus 2 Cellular Complex Blend Capsules 2 times daily. Or 1-5 drops Topical Blend, Melaleuca, Outdoor Blend or Protective Blend to area.

Lavender with any oils gives additional soothing relief.

Other oils: Eucalyptus^EC, Geranium^EC, Lemon^EC, Rosemary^EC

Parkinson's disease   *see also* Essential tremors

Oils: Frankincense^C **Blends/Products:** Basic Vitality Supplements, Grounding Blend^C, Massage Blend

1-2 drops Frankincense under tongue and 1-2 drops along spine daily, Basic Vitality Supplements consistently and the Massage Blend Technique at least weekly.

Agitation/frustration: Hand massage or diffuse Grounding Blend, Lavender or Restful Blend. *see also* Irritability.

Other oils: Ginger[C], Lavender[C], Myrrh[C], Peppermint[C], Ylang Ylang[C]
Blends: Restful Blend[C]

Passion   *see* Emotional strength

Patchouli *(Pogostemon cablin)*

essential&oil

Properties: Antibiotic, antidepressant, antifungal, anti-inflammatory, antiseptic, antitoxic, astringent, decongestant, diuretic, sedative

Addresses: Acne, ADHD, Alzheimer's, anxiety, autism, breathing disorders, deodorant, depression, dermatitis, eczema, hemorrhoids, insect bites, scarring, skin care, snake bites, stress, stroke, wounds

PCOS *(polycystic ovary syndrome)*

Oils: Basil, Clary Sage, Frankincense **Blends:** Monthly Blend for Women, Phytoestrogen Complex

Root cause: *see* Hormonal balance for more on Phytoestrogen Complex and Monthly Blend for Women that are specifically formulated to balance hormones and manage menstrual problems.

Also consider: 2-3 drops Frankincense under tongue every night and morning.

Or: 8 drops each Clary Sage, Frankincense, Lavender, Cypress, 2 Tbsp melted VCO; soak tampon in mixture, insert overnight nightly for one week. Switch to 8 drops each Frankincense, Geranium, 5 drops Myrrh, 2 Tbsp grape seed oil.

Pain/Cramps: Soothing Blend or Basil with Clary Sage

Other oils: Cypress, Geranium, Helichrysum, Lavender, Myrrh **Blends:** Soothing Blend

Legend: Preferred, Suggested, Consider

Peaceful Child Blend

Ingredients: Clary Sage, Frankincense, Lavender, Marjoram, Vetiver, Ylang Ylang with FCO (available on line, search for PeacefulChildBlend)

Addresses: ADD/ADHD, Autism, Asperger's, Schizophrenia, Sensory Processing Disorder (SPD), Tourette syndrome

(see Safety Chart, page 23)

Pelvic pain syndrome   *see also* Prostate conditions

Oils: Helichrysum, Frankincense, White Fir, Wintergreen **Blends:** Grounding Blend, Massage Blend

If possible identify root cause and use protocol suggested for this elsewhere in this book.

Chronic pain: 2-3 drops Wintergreen and Frankincense or White Fir and Helichrysum with 5-10 drops FCO and massage into area 2x daily. Also consider the Massage Blend Technique periodically.

Other oils: Lemongrass, Lavender[C], Melaleuca, Peppermint, Wild Orange **Blends:** Soothing Blend

Peppermint *(Mentha piperita)*

(also available in a roll-on)

Properties: Analgesic, anti-inflammatory, antiparasitic, antiseptic, antispasmodic, astringent, expectorant, stimulant

Addresses: Allergies, asthma, bronchitis, cold and flu, colic, congestion, dermatitis, diarrhea, fever, headaches, indigestion, insect bites, insect repellent, menstrual problems, mental acuity, migraines, motion sickness, nausea, skin disorders, stomachache, stress, toothache

(see Safety Chart, page 23)

Peppermint products

essentialōoils
Product

Roll-on: Provides gentle and convenient application.

Beadlets: Convenient soft vegetarian beadlets that quickly dissolves in the mouth and invigorates the senses. Can be used for oral care, respiratory health, digestive comfort and other internal uses for Peppermint.

(see Safety Chart, page 23)

Peptic ulcer   *see* Ulcers

Pericarditis *(inflammation of surrounding sac)*   *see* Heart conditions

Perimenopause   *see* Menopause

Periodontal disease   *see* Gum conditions

Peripheral artery disease (PAD)   *see* Heart conditions

Periungual warts   *see* Warts

Personal care *(Hand & Body)*   *see also* Skin care (facial), Hair care

essentialōoils
Product

Products for a variaty of personal care needs based on essential oils can be a great asset. A number are shown below.

HAND & BODY CLEANSING

Bath Bars:

> **Moisturizing:** A natural bar that leaves the skin feeling clean, smooth and soft with the soothing fragrance of Bergamot and Grapefruit essential oils.

> **Invigorating:** This bar provides an invigorating cleansing expereince with this uplifting blend.

> **Restful:** This is a one-of-a-kind bar that provides a unique feel, lather, aroma and cleansing experience. Infused with the unique Restful Blend.

Legend: Preferred, Suggested, Consider

Refreshing Body Wash: The refreshing scents of Bergamot, Cedarwood and Grapefruit make using this wash a pleasant way to start the day.

Exfoliating Body Scrub: A body scrub with natural sugar cane to gently exfoliate and polish the skin. To this is added the essential oils of Ginger, Grapefruit and Wild Orange plus kukui, macadamia and coconut oils for a unique at-home experience.

HAND & BODY LOTIONS

Invigorating (Citrus) Hand Lotion: This beautiful lotions combines the essential oils of Clementine peel, Grapefruit, Lemon, Mandarin peel, Tangerine peel, Vanilla bean absolute, Wild Orange (a popular citrus blend) with hydrating seed oils and nourishing botanicals.

Rose Hand Lotion: Rose essential oil is known for its benefits to skin care and is combined with natural moisturizers and humectants for a lotion that promotes smooth, beautiful skin.

Hand & Body Lotion: A lotion with a base of jojoba and macadamia seed oils with murumuru and theobroma seed butters plus nourishing plant extracts. To this can be added the essential oils of choice to make a personal quality lotion.

Replenishing Body Butter: For areas requiring intense moisturizing (elbows, hands, knees) this formulation of Douglas Fir, Frankincense and Wild Orange essential oils combined with shea and cocoa seed butters plus jojoba seed oils and avocado oil provides an exceptional and unique solution.

HAND & BODY OTHER HELPS

Natural Deodorant: Bergamot, Cedarwood, Cypress and Melaleuca essential oils are infused into a natural formula giving an odor-fighting product for men and women.

Lip Balm: Essential oils combined with coconut, moringa seed and avocado oils with beeswax gives a lip balm that soothes and hydrates. Three essential oils combinations provide three unique flavors:
>   Original: Peppermint and Wild Orange
>   Tropical: Clementine, Lime and Ylang Ylang
>   Herbal: Lemon Verbena, Marjoram and Spearmint

Safety charts ... page 23   Special cautions ... page 3   223

Personality disorders *see also* Emotional conditions and Mental conditions

[OCD (Obsessive compulsive disorder), Paranoia, Schizophrenia]

Alzheimer's	*see* Alzheimer's
Bipolar (manic depression)	*see* Bipolar
Dementia	*see* Dementia
OCD (obsessive compulsive disorder)	*see* Obsessive compulsive disorder
Paranoia	*see* Paranoia
Postpartum depression	*see* Pregnancy
PTSD (post traumatic stress disorder)	*see* Stress
Schizophrenia	*see* Schizophrenia

Perspiration, excess *see* Body odor

Pets *see* Animals

Petitgrain *(Citrus x aurantium)*

essential **oil**

Properties: Antispasmodic, antidepressant, anti-inflammatory, antioxidant, antiseptic, calming, sedative, uplifting

Addresses: Acne, anxiety, body odor , cough (spasmodic), dandruff, depression, excess perspiration, fatigue, flatulence, indigestion, inflammation, insomnia, irritability, mental confussion, mental fatigue, mood swings, muscle spasms, oily hair, stress

(see Safety Chart, page 23)

Phenols *see* Chemical constituents

Phlebitis *see* Blood clots

Phytoestrogen Complex *(Women's Phytoestrogen Complex)*

essential **oils**
Product

Hormone balance supplement

The Phytoestrogen Complex is a blend of natural plant extracts that support hormone balance throughout the different phases of a women's life. Balancing hormones and managing harmful

Legend: Preferred, Suggested, Consider

metabolites by eating a healthy diet rich in phytoestrogens and other essential nutrients, exercising and managing weight can help reduce uncomfortable symptoms associated with PMS and the transition through menopause and supports healthy bones, heart, breast tissue and other body structures and functions as a women ages.

Pimples
see Acne

Pink eye
see Conjunctivitis

Pink Pepper *(Schinus molle)*

essential oil

Properties: Analgesic, antibacterial, antifungal, anti-inflammatory, antimicrobial, antiseptic, antispasmodic, antitumoral, antiviral, astringent, calming, digestive, diuretic, stimulant (digestive)

Addresses: Arthritis, candida, cuts & wounds, digestive problems, fatigue (energizing), muscle pain, restlessness (calming)

(see Safety Chart, page 23)

Plaque
see Gum conditions

Plantar fasciitis

Oils: Lemongrass **Blends:** Soothing Blend

Soothing Blend Rub with 2-4 drops Lemongrass topically to bottom of foot and calf of leg and follow with warm compress before retiring. Same oils first thing in morning coupled with sitting and bending toes forward and backward. If severe apply oils during day.

Alternative oil combinations: Lemongrass/Peppermint/Wintergreen or Helichrysum/Peppermint.

Other oils: Basil, Birch, Cypress, Frankincense, Helichrysum, Peppermint, Wintergreen

Plantar warts
see Warts

Pleurisy

Oils: Cypress[C], Thyme[C] **Blends:** Respiratory Blend

2-3 drops Cypress and Thyme applied topically to the painful area of chest 2-3x daily. Cup & inhale and/or diffuse Respiratory Blend (or Cypress and Thyme) 2-3x daily.

Severe: With Respiratory Blend cup & inhale slowly and as deeply as possible every 2 hours. Diffuse Respiratory Blend as much as possible. On the chest area layer Cypress and Thyme (with carrier oil for skin sensitivity) and add Peppermint to drive first oils deeper. Repeat 2-3 times daily. For additional support some suggest also taking capsules with 4 drops Protective Blend and 3 drops of Oregano and/or Thyme 2-3 times daily. The latter is a strong use of essential oils. Only consider for adults without sensitivities.

Ongoing: Use Lemon water often, Basic Vitality Supplements, GI Cleansing Formula/Probiotic Defense Formula cleanses and a healthy diet.

Other oils: Basil, Bergamot, Frankincense, Lemon, Melaleuca, Oregano, Peppermint, Roman Chamomile **Blends/Products:** Basic Vitality Supplements, GI Cleansing Formula/Probiotic Defense Formula, Protective Blend

PMS (premenstrual syndrome)

see also Acne, Depression, Hormonal balance, Mood swings
[Anger, Acne, Anxiety, Cramps, Depression, Disinterest, Irritability]

Oils: Lavender, Melaleuca, Sandalwood[C] **Blends/Products:** Basic Vitality Supplements, Blend for Women, Massage Blend, Monthly Blend for Women, Phytoestrogen Complex, Restful Blend[C], Soothing Blend, Tension Blend[C]

Prevention: Basic Vitality Supplements and Phytoestrogen Complex consistently (*see* Hormone balance)

Symptom relief: 2-4 drops Monthly Blend for Women topically to abdomen as needed for discomfort with warm compress, also consider the Massage Blend Technique periodically.

Additional help:
    Cramps: 2-4 drops Monthly Blend for Women or Tension Blend

topically to abdomen with warm compress or 8-12 drops Sandalwood in capsule at outset then second day 6-8 drops and/or Soothing Blend to lower abdomen and lower back.

Anger, anxiety, disinterest: 2-3 drops Restful Blend or Blend for Women to bottoms of feet, back of neck and/or diffuse.

Acne: Lavender and Melaleuca topically.

Other oils: Cypress, Frankincense, Geranium[C], Helichrysum, Neroli[EC], Rosemary, Spikenard, Yarrow[C], Ylang Ylang[C] **Blends:** Cleansing Blend, Grounding Blend[C], Topical Blend

Pneumonia

Oils: Frankincense[C], Lavender[EC], Lemon[EC], Melaleuca[C], Oregano[C], Peppermint **Blends:** Protective Blend[C], Respiratory Blend

4 drops Protective Blend, 3 drops each Frankincense and Oregano on bottoms of feet or in capsule with FCO 3x daily. Diffuse or cup & inhale Respiratory Blend often. Gargle and oil pull Oregano (hot/dilute) and Lemon in drinking water. Add 1-3 drops Lemon and Peppermint to water, drink lots. Also consider the Massage Blend Technique periodically and/or blend above in a capsule as suppository or with enema.

Children: 1 drops each Frankincense, Lavender, Melaleuca on bottoms of feet, diffuse or steam tent with Respiratory Blend.

Other oils: Basil, Cinnamon Bark[C], Cypress[C], Eucaplyptus[EC], Rosemary, Thyme[C]

Note: When choosing alternative oils from the list of "**Other oils:**" please review safety precautions on pages 23-28.

Poison ivy

[poison oak, poison sumac]

Oils: Frankincense, Myrrh, Peppermint **Blends:** Protective Blend

2-4 drops Peppermint and Protective Blend (or Frankincense, Myrrh) directly to area. If too sensitive to touch use spray bottle. At least 3x daily.

Other oils: Birch, Eucalyptus[C], Lavender[C], Roman Chamomile[C], Rose[C]

Polycystic ovary syndrome   *see* PCOS

Polymyalgia rheumatica
see Muscle cramps

Polyps
see also Tumor

Frankincense[C], Melaleuca

Nasal: 1-3 drops Frankincense to bridge of nose; with Q-tips gently in nostril; under tongue or in capsule 1-2x daily.

Other: 1-3 drops Frankincense under tongue or capsule 1-2x daily.

Other oils: Basil[C], Oregano[C], Peppermint[C] **Blends:** Cleansing Blend[C], Grounding Blend[C]

Pore reduction
see Personal care and Skin care

Post nasal drip
see Colds

Post traumatic stress disorder (PTSD)
see Stress

Postpartum depression
see Pregnancy

Pregnancy
see also Breastfeeding, Childbirth

The following is a brief summary of suggestions during pregnancy. The book *Essential Oils for Pregnancy, Birth and Babies* is an excellent, more complete, resource. Be aware this summary does not include all cautions one should be aware of during pregnancy and we advise reading the cautions regarding pregnancy for any oil recommended. See pages 19-29.

Back pain

Oils: Lavender[C], Marjoram[C] **Blends:** Massage Blend[C], Soothing Blend[C]

Massage area with Massage Blend, Soothing Blend, Lavender or Marjoram.

Bleeding

Bleeding during pregnancy can be serious, seeking professional medical counsel is advised.

Breast, tender

Legend: Preferred, Suggested, Consider

Oils: Geranium[C], Lavender[C], Roman Chamomile[C] **Blends:** Monthly Blend for Women[C]

Topical application of Monthly Blend for Women or oils above singly or in blend with FCO.

Breastfeeding (lactation, nursing)   *see* Breastfeeding

Calming

Oils: Lavender[C], Frankincense[C], Ylang Ylang[C] **Blends:** Grounding Blend[C], Restful Blend[C]

Any of above oils and blends diffuse, cup & inhale or 3-5 drops in warm bath.

Constipation

Oils: Coriander[C], Ginger[C], Peppermint[C] **Blends:** Digestive Blend[C]

1-3 drops of one of above topically to abdomen in circular motions moving up from right side or internally in capsule or with tsp honey and tea.

Delivery   *see* Childbirth

Edema (swelling)

Oils: Cypress[C], Ginger[C], Lavender[C], Lemon[C] **Blends:** Massage Blend[C]

Blend 5 drops each Massage Blend, Cypress, 2 drops each Ginger, Lavender, Lemon, 1 Tbsp FCO; massage feet and legs starting with feet (hands) with movements towards heart.

Fatigue

Oils: Coriander[C], Grapefruit[C], Lavender[C], Peppermint[C], Rosemary[C] **Blends:** Invigorating Blend[C], Joyful Blend[C]

Invigorating Blend, Joyful Blend or blend of equal parts Coriander, Grapefruit, Lavender. Diffuse, cup & inhale, with FCO massage neck and shoulders.

Heartburn or indigestion   *see also* Heartburn
Oils: Ginger^C, Peppermint^C **Blends:** Digestive Blend^C, Invigorating Blend^C

1-2 drops of above topically to abdomen or internally in capsule.

Hemorrhoids   *see also* Hemorrhoids
Oils: Cypress^C, Geranium^C, Helichrysum^C, Lavender^C

Blend equal parts Cypress, Geranium, Lavender or Cypress and Helichrysum topically with FCO if preferred.

Labor   *see* Childbirth

Leg (muscle) cramps
Oils: Cypress^C, Geranium^C, Lavender^C **Blends:** Massage Blend^C

2-4 drops Massage Blend or blend of 5 drops Cypress, Geranium, 10 drops Lavender, 2 Tbsp FCO topically to area.

Miscarriage, after a
Oils: Clary Sage^C, Geranium^C, Lavender^C

Support physically and emotionally with a blend of above oils.

Morning sickness
Oils: Coriander^C, Ginger^C, Peppermint^C **Blends:** Digestive Blend^C

1-3 drops of one of above topically on abdomen, in a capsule or sipped with water or juice.

Nutrition
Blends/Products: Basic Vitality Supplements^C, Bone Nutrient Complex^C, Probiotic Defense Formula^C

Natural whole foods with consistent use of supplements above is very important. Avoid sugars, sodas and refined grains.

Postpartum depression   *see* Childbirth

Stretch marks   *see also* Stretch marks
Oils: Frankincense^C, Geranium^C, Grapefruit^C, Helichrysum^C, Lavender^C **Blends/Products:** Anti-Aging Blend^C, Anti-Aging Moisturizer, Hand & Body Lotion^C (*see* Skin care)

Apply moisturizing skin lotion topically with Anti-Aging Blend or Hand & Body Lotion with oils above and use in areas with potential for stretch marks before they occur. Apply 2-3x daily.

Varicose veins   *see also* Varicose veins

Oils: Cypress[C], Geranium[C], Helichrysum[C], Lavender[C]

Blend 15 drops each Geranium, Lavender (optional), 5 drops each Cypress and Helichrysum, 1 Tbsp VCO, topically apply with gentle strokes from ankles to thighs with motion towards the heart.

Premenopause   *see* Menopause

Premenstrual syndrome   *see* PMS

Presbyopia   *see* Eyesight failing

Pressure ulcers   *see* Bedsores

Probiotic Defense Formula   *see also* Supplements

essential●oils
Product

Probiotics Defense Formula: This is a blend of pre-biotic fiber and six strains of probiotic microorganisms in a unique double-layer vegetable capsule delivering 5 billion CFUs of active probiotic cultures and soluble pre-biotic FOS (fructo-oligosaccharides) that encourages culture adhesion and growth. This supports healthy digestive functions, immunities and is safe for use by all ages.

Powdered Probiotic: Probiotics are also available in a powder sachet so the tasty powder can be poured directly in the mouth. Perfect for children and those with swallowing difficulties.

Prostate conditions   *see also* Cancer

[BPH (benign prostatic hypertrophy), pelvic pain syndrome, prostatitis]

Oils: Clove[C], Frankincense[C], Lavender[C], Thyme[C] **Blends:** Invigorating Blend[C]

BPH: 3 drops each Invigorating Blend, Frankincense, 2 drops each Clove, Lavender, Thyme in capsule orally 2-3x daily or rectal with rectal

---

retention nightly.

Other oils: Cypress[C], Myrrh, Oregano, Yarrow[C]

Note: When choosing alternative oils from the list of "**Other oils:**" please review safety precautions on pages 23-28.

Protective Blend *(guards from pathogens)*

Ingredients: Cinnamon Bark, Clove bud, Eucalyptus, Rosemary, Wild Orange

Another common formulation: Clove, Lemon, Cinnamon Bark, Eucalyptus radiata and Rosemary

Addresses: Bacteria, immune system support, mold, topical disinfectant, virus

(see Safety Chart, page 23)

Protective Blend for Children   *see* Kid's Blends

Protective Blend products

essential oils
Product

Personal products:

Roll-on: Provides gentle and convenient application.

Beadlets: Tiny vegetable beadlets that freshens breath and supports the immune system.

Softgels: see Protective Blend+ below

Throat Drops: Protective Blend in a natural, convenient tasty throat drop to calm dry, scratchy throats.

Mouthwash: Daily rinse cleans teeth and gums, reduces plaque and freshens breath.

Natural Whitening Toothpaste: The Protective Blend adds a cleansing boost to other natural cleaning ingredients.

(see Safety Chart, page 23)

Handy household cleansing products:

Foaming Hand Wash: In easy to use pump dispensers provides a gentle, natural, convenient cleanser.

Hand Sanitizing Spray: Protective Blend allowing

Legend: Preferred, Suggested, Consider

convenient, no rinse protection from germs and bacteria.

Laundry Detergent: Protective Blend with bio-originated enzymes to clean and lift laundry stains.

Cleaner Concentrate: Ideal for cleaning and sanitizing living spaces with a natural cleaner.

Protective Blend+ *(in a softgel)*

Product

The Protective Blend (Cinnamon Bark, Clove bud, Eucalyptus, Rosemary, Wild Orange) plus Black Pepper, Melissa and Oregano for additional immune support. Packaged in a vegetarian softgel delivery system for ease.

(see Safety Chart, page 23)

Psoriasis
see also Eczema

Oils: Geranium[EC], Lavender[EC], Melaleuca[C] **Blends:** Topical Blend[C]

Topical Blend or self-made blend using 10 drops Lavender, 5 drops each Helichrysum and Myrrh, 3-5 drops Melaleuca with 1 tsp EVCO. Apply topically to area.

Cleanses: GI Cleansing Formula/Probiotic Defense Formula, Detoxification Blend or 2-3 drops Lemon with each glass of water.

Basic Vitality Supplements on a consistent basis.

Other oils: Arborvitae[C], Cedarwood[C], Copaiba[C], Frankincense[C], Grapefruit, Helichrysum[C], Lemon, Myrrh, Roman Chamomile[EC]

Psychological disorders
see Personality disorders

PTSD *(post traumatic stress disorder)*
see Stress

Puerperal infection *(childbirth fever)*
see Pregnancy

Pulling, oil
see Oil Pulling

Pus
see Infections

Pyelonephritis
see Kidney infection

Notes:

Legend: Preferred, Suggested, Consider

Rabies

see Animal bites

Rashes

see also Detoxification, Eczema, Impetigo, Insect bites, Parasite infections, Poison Ivy, Scabies

Oils: Lavender[C], Melaleuca[C], Spikenard[C] **Blends:** Cleansing Blend[C], Digestive Enzyme Complex[C]

Address root cause, see list of possibilities above under *see also*.

General helps:

Topical: Lavender applied neat to area (or other oils above).

Internal: 3-4 Digestive Enzyme Complex capsules 3x daily, Basic Vitality Supplements and GI Cleansing Formula/Probiotic Defense Formula cleanse.

Other oils: Elemi[C], Manuka[C], Myrrh[EC], Roman Chamomile[EC], Sandalwood[EC]

Ravensara *(Ravensara aromaticum)*

essential oil

Properties: Analgesic, antibacterial, antidepressant, antifungal, anti-infectious, anti-inflammatory, antiseptic, antiviral, calming, decongestant, expectorant, sedative

Addresses: Bronchitis, colds, cough, depression, fatigue, flu, hepatitis, muscle pain, shingles, sinus infection, viral infection, whooping cough

Artistically created. Essential Oils Books

Raynaud's disease

Circulation: Oils: Cypress
Stress: Oils: Patchouli Blends: Grounding Blend

Improve circulation by applying 1-3 drops Cypress with 10 drops carrier to area. For stress inhale Grounding Blend as needed.

Other oils:
>**Circulation:** Geranium, Helichrysum
>**Stress:** Blends: Restful Blend, Tension Blend

Reassuring Blend

essential oils
Blend

(comes in a roll-on dispenser)

Ingredients: Clary Sage, Frankincense, Labdanum, Lavender, Marjoram, Spearmint, Vetiver, Ylang Ylang

Addresses: An emotional health blend to bring peace and calm in troubling occasions.

(see Safety Chart, page 23)

Reflexology points

Definition Points on feet, hands or ears identified in some alternative health techniques as being connected to vital organs and other locations on the body. Oils are applied to specific reflexology points to deliver their benefits to the vital organ or other body locations. See the Helpful Charts section at the end of this book for more details.

Relaxing   see Anxiety

Renal failure   see Kidney failure

Renewing Blend

essential oils
Blend

(comes in a roll-on dispenser)

Ingredients: Arborvitae, Bergamot, Citronella, Juniper Berry, Myrrh, Nootka Tree, Spruce, Thyme

Addresses: An emotional health blend to strengthen forgiveness and renew the spirit after disappointment.

(see Safety Chart, page 23)

Repellent Blend   see Outdoor Blend

Legend: Preferred, Suggested, Consider

Respiratory Blend *(breathe better)*

essential oils
Blend

Ingredients: Cardamom, Eucalyptus, Laurel leaf, Lemon, Melaleuca, Peppermint, Ravensara leaf

Other common formulations: Eucalyptus Radiata, Lemon, Peppermint, Ravensara, Wintergreen

And: Cypress, Eucalyptus, Eucalyptus Citriodora, Eucalyptus Radiata, Lavender, Marjoram, Myrtus, Peppermint, Pine, Tsuga

Addresses: Asthma, bronchitis, cold and flu, congestion, cough, respiratory stress

(see Safety Chart, page 23)

Respiratory Blend products

essential oils
Blend

Roll-on: Gentle and quick application.

Vapor Stick: Smooth, convenient and quick application.

Throat drops: Great tasting, convenient longenges.

(see Safety Chart, page 23)

Respiratory conditions

Acute bronchitis	*see* Bronchitis
Asthma	*see* Asthma
Chronic bronchitis	*see* Bronchitis
COPD (Chronic obstructive pulmonary disease)	*see* COPD
Cystic fibrosis	*see* Cystic fibrosis
Emphysema	*see* Emphysema
Lung cancer	*see* Cancer
Pleurisy	*see* Pleurisy
Pneumonia	*see* Pneumonia
RSV (respiratory syncytial virus)	*see* RSV
Tuberculosis	*see* Tuberculosis

Restful Blend *(can help give a serene attitude)*

essential●oils (also available in Softgels and a Bath Bar)

Blend

Ingredients: Cedarwood, Ho Wood, Lavender, Roman Chamomile, Sandalwood (Hawaiian), Sweet Marjoram leaf, Vanilla bean absolute, Vetiver, Ylang Ylang

Another common formulation: Blue Tansy, Orange, Patchouli, Tangerine, Ylang Ylang

Addresses: Anxiety, calming, induces restfulness and restful sleep, soothing, stress (use softgel for restful night's sleep)

(see Safety Chart, page 23)

Restful Blend for Children   *see* Kid's Blends

Restless leg syndrome *(RLS)*

Blends/Products: Massage Blend, Soothing Blend^C

2-4 drops Massage Blend massaged into area as episode begins. Use carrier to help massage. Also consider Soothing Blend or other oils with same massage application.

Other oils: Marjoram^C, Roman Chamomile **Blends:** Restful Blend

Restlessness   *see* Anxiety

Retinal detachment   *see* Eyesight failing

Rheumatic fever

Oils: Frankincense, Ginger^C, Myrrh **Blends/Products:** Detoxification Blend, Respiratory Blend, Soothing Blend, Basic Vitality Supplements, GI Cleansing Formula/Probiotic Defense Formula, Detoxification Complex

To help with pain symptoms: Rub Soothing Blend topically on the affected limbs and joints. Respiratory Blend if there is shortness of breath.

To help long term: Detoxify the cleansing organs with Detoxification Complex: 2 tablets daily, 1 morning, 1 evening. 5 drops of the Detoxification Blend in a capsule daily. Continue this consistently. Also follow the Gastrointestinal tract cleanse described under Detoxification.

Smaller children: Cut open GI Cleansing Formula and Detoxification Blend capsules and apply oils to bottoms of the feet. Scale based on the size of the child.

Some suggest applying 1 - 3 drops of Frankincense and Myrrh daily to lymph nodes to assist cleansing process.

Other oils: Rosemary

Rheumatism
see Arthritis

Rheumatoid arthritis
see Arthritis

Rhinitis (stuffy nose)
see Allergies or Colds

Ringing in ears
see Tinnitis

Ringworm

Oils: Lavender^C, Melaleuca^C, Thyme^C **Blends:** Topical Blend^C

Topical Blend or make blend with equal parts Lavender, Melaleuca and Thyme. 2-3 drops of either blend (with carrier if needed) on area of infection 3x daily for 10 days. Follow with Melaleuca (may be mixed 3:1 with carrier oil) for 30 days to assure fungus does not return. Also consider Cellular Complex Blend topically to area and 2 Cellular Complex Blend caplets 2x daily.

Additional itching relief: Lavender topically

Other oils: Geranium^{EC}, Neroli^C, Oregano^C, Peppermint^{EC} **Blends:** Cellular Complex Blend^C

RLS
see Restless leg syndrome

Roller bottle

Deinition An application technique wherein an oil or blend with or without a carrier is added to an empty bottle with a roller dispenser top (commercially available) for easy, handy topical application of the oil or blend.

Roman Chamomile *(Anthemis nobilis)*

essential oil

Properties: Antibacterial, antidepressant, anti-inflammatory, antiparasitic, antispasmodic, antiviral

Addresses: Acne, allergies, anxiety, depression, earache, fever, mental acuity, stomachache, stress, teething pain

(see Safety Chart, page 23)

Rosacea

Blends/Products: Detoxification Blend, Detoxification Complex, GI Cleansing Formula/ Probiotic Defense Formula, Topical Blend

May be autoimmune or infectious, consider both approaches simultaneously. Use Basic Vitality Supplements consistently.

Autoimmune, mild detox: 2 tablets Detoxification Complex and 5 drops Detoxification Blend in capsule daily.

Autoimmune, aggressive detox: 3 capsules GI Cleansing Formula daily with meals, 10 days (adjust number for age and sensitivity). Then 3 capsules Probiotic Defense Formula daily with meals, 5 days. Rest 10-15 days, repeat 2x. Some find GI Cleansing Formula detox eliminates toxins so rapidly that it stresses skin. If so, reduce GI Cleansing Formula to 1 or 2 capsules per day or use only Detoxification Blend detoxification.

Infectious: 2-5 drops Topical Blend apply morning and night topically on area. (Or self-made blend with oils below.)

Other oils: Frankincense, Helichrysum[C], Lavender[C], Rosemary[C], Sandalwood[C] **Blends/Products:** Basic Vitality Supplements

Rose *(Rosa damascena)*

essential oil

(comes in a roll-on and Hand Lotion)

Properties: Antibacterial, Antidepressant, Antihemorrhaging, Anti-inflammatory, Antispasmodic, Antiviral, aphrodisiac, astringent, emmenagogue, laxative, stomachic

Legend: Preferred, Suggested, Consider

Addresses: Depression, digestive disorders, hemorrhaging, menstrual problems, postpartum depression, uplifting

(see Safety Chart, page 23)

Rosemary *(Rosmarinus officinalis)*

essential oil

Properties: Analgesic, antioxidant, antiseptic, antispasmodic, astringent, diuretic, stimulant

Addresses: Arthritic pain, asthma, bronchitis, cold and flu, constipation, dermatitis, diarrhea, gout, hypotension, indigestion, menstrual problems, migraines, muscle pain, skin disorders, stress, stomachache

(see Safety Chart, page 23)

RSV *(respiratory syncytial virus)*

Oils: Basil, Lime, Rosemary **Blends:** Respiratory Blend

Dilute one of the blends below 2:1 with FCO:
  Respiratory Blend
  Basil, Lime and Rosemary
  10 drops each Respiratory Blend and Lime, 5 drops Frankincense, 2 drops Oregano, 1 drop Thyme.

All: Apply to bottoms of feet every 1-2 hours and diffuse Respiratory Blend.

Babies: Cover with socks to prevent transfer of oils to eyes.

Older children/adults: Apply oil blend to chest area also.

To calm: Use Grounding Blend[c] or Lavender.

Other oils: Eucalyptus[c], Frankincense, Oregano, Thyme

Rubella   *see* German measles

Rubeola   *see* Measles

Notes:

Legend: Preferred, Suggested, Consider

Sadness   *see* Anxiety

Safety   *see* Safety Considerations section at front of book

Salmonella   *see* Food poisoning

Sandalwood, Indian *(Santalum album)*

essential oil

Sandalwood, Hawaiian *Santalum panicuatum*

Note: Sandalwood and Hawaiian Sandalwood are very similar in constituents and can be used interchangeably.

Properties: Antibacterial, antidepressant, antifungal, anti-inflammatory, antiseptic, aphrodisiac, carminative, disinfectant, diuretic, expectorant, sedative, stimulant

Addresses: Acne, asthma, bronchitis, candida, dermatitis, cold and flu, cough, skin disorders, stress, throat infections, yeast infections

Scabies

Oils: Melaleuca[C], Oregano **Blends/Products:** Cellular Complex Blend[C], Cleansing Blend, Protective Blend[C], Soothing Blend Rub[C]

Equal parts Cellular Complex Blend and Soothing Blend Rub topically to area 3-4x daily. For increased help add 2 Cellular Complex Blend caplets 2x daily.

Alternative: Equal parts Melaleuca or Cleansing Blend and carrier in glass spray bottle applied 2-3x daily. If more difficult add Oregano with additional carrier oil to spray.

Prevent spreading: Cleanse areas touched with Protective Blend.

Other oils: Bergamot[EC], Lavender[EC], Peppermint[EC] **Blends:** Outdoor Blend, Topical Blend[C]

Scar reduction

Oils: Frankincense^C, Helichrysum^{EC}, Lavender^C

6 drops each Helichrysum, Frankincense and Lavender, plus Vitamin E oil from 6 capsules and 10 Tbsp EVCO or other carrier for ointment to apply to area 2-3x daily.

Other oils: Copaiba^C, Geranium^C, Jasmine^C, Myrrh^C, Neroli^C, Rose^C, Yarrow^C

Schizophrenia   *see also* Personality disorders

Oils: Vetiver **Blends:** Grounding Blend

1-2 drops Grounding Blend or Vetiver in roller bottle, apply behind ears, on wrists, bottoms of feet and/or along spine 2-3x daily. Also diffuse or cup & inhale.

Other oils: Frankincense, Lavender **Blends:** Monthly Blend for Women, Peaceful Child Blend

Schmidt's syndrome   *see* Adrenal conditions

Sciatica   *see also* Back conditions

Oils: Cypress^C, Helichrysum^C, Myrrh^C **Blends/Products:** Massage Blend, Soothing Blend^C

Use the Massage Blend Technique at least daily, follow with hot compress. Sciatic nerve starts in lower back, L4, L5, and S1 then thru hip and down back of legs. Nerve pressure and pain can occur anywhere on path. Nerve pressure often compounded with other problems noted below, supplement the Massage Blend Technique with any or all of these:

Immediate pain relief:· Soothing Blend or Soothing Blend Rub. Also consider Birch or Wintergreen. 2 -3 drops topically to area of pain as needed.

Reduce inflammation: Myrrh or also consider Bergamot, Black Pepper, Roman Chamomile or Rosemary. 2-3 drops topically where nerve is being pinched 2-3x daily.

Legend: Preferred, Suggested, Consider

Relax muscles/spasms: Massage Blend or also consider Lavender, Marjoram or Melissa. 2-3 drops to area where spasm is occurring.

Increase circulation: Cypress or also consider Invigorating Blend, Eucalyptus, Geranium, Lemon or Peppermint. 2-3 drops to spinal area 2-3x per day.

Encourage helping and tissue regeneration: Helichrysum or also consider Frankincense or Sandalwood. 1-2 drops topically to spinal area 2-3x per day followed by hot compress.

Also use: Diffuse and/or baths with 4-5 drops relaxing oils.

Other oils: Bergamot, Black Pepper, Birch, Eucalyptus, Frankincense[C], Geranium[C], Lavender, Lemon[C], Marjoram, Melissa, Peppermint[C], Sandalwood[C], White Fir[C], Wintergreen **Blends:** Grounding Blend[C], Invigorating Blend

Scleroderma   see also Autoimmune diseases

Oils: Frankincense[C], Lemongrass **Blends/Products:** Basic Vitality Supplements, Cellular Complex Blend, Soothing Blend

Consistent Basic Vitality Supplements, 8 drops or 1 capsule Cellular Complex Blend 2x daily. 2-3 drops Frankincense 2-4x daily under tongue or internally.

Symptoms: 2-3 drops Lemongrass with Soothing Blend Rub to affected area. Also 4 drops each Myrrh and Sandalwood to bottoms of feet and along spine, rotate with 3 drops each Birch, Soothing Blend and Lavender.

Other oils: Basil[C], Birch, Geranium[C], Lavender, Lemon[C], Myrrh, Sandalwood, Wild Orange[C]

Scoliosis   see also Back conditions, Sciatica

The Massage Blend Technique is recommended daily and consistently:
        Stress management: Grounding Blend, Lavender
        Immune support: Melaleuca, Protective Blend
        Inflammatory response: Massage Blend, Soothing Blend
        Homeostasis: Peppermint, Wild Orange

Peppermint (last step): For some this is too cool/stimulating. Reduce to 1-2 drops.

Smaller children: Same oils, same order, fewer drops with carrier oil or only on bottoms of feet.

Self apply: No one to do the Massage Blend Technique? Use the same oils, same order, self apply to feet and on spine as far as able to reach.

Other oils: Frankincense, Marjoram **Blends:** Soothing Blend

Scrapes   *see also* Cuts and wounds

Oils: Frankincense[EC], Helichrysum[EC], Lavender[EC], Melaleuca[EC], Myrrh[EC]
Blends: Protective Blend[C]

Minor scrapes: Apply Lavender neat topically.

More serious scrapes and road rashes:

Cleansing: Remove debris, then use Protective Blend Foaming Wash and follow with an Protective Blend spritz.

Antibiotic: Topical apply Lavender, Frankincense or Myrrh.

Pain relief, calming: Apply Lavender neat to wound, for a child rub palms together with 2-3 drops of oil and let child inhale.

Ongoing: Repeat application of antibiotic oil every 4-6 hours. Apply Helichrysum during process and to reduce scarring.

Other oils: Blue Tansy[C], Copiaba[C], Lemon[C], Manuka[C], Ravensara[C], Yarrow[C]

Sea sick   *see* Motion sickness

Seasonal Blend in a softgel *(three oils to ease allergies)*

essential oils
Blend

Ingredients: A softgel each with 2 drops of Lavender, Lemon, Peppermint.

Addresses: Protection against seasonal and environmental elements and promotes a healthy respiratory system.

(see Safety Chart, page 23)

Legend: Preferred, Suggested, Consider

Sebaceous cyst   *see also* Cysts

Oils: Frankincense

2-3 drops topically, 1-2x daily until gone.

Other oils: Lavender, Lemongrass, Topical Blend **Blends:** Massage Blend

Sedative   *see* Insomnia

Seizures   *see also* Epilepsy

Oils: Frankincense[c] **Blends:** Grounding Blend[c]

ATTENTION: Seizures can be a symptom of a very serious medical condition and should have immediate attention with professional medical help.

Preventive help: 2-3 drops Grounding Blend and Frankincense to bottoms of feet, brain stem and back of head daily.

Basic Vitality Supplements and Massage Blend Technique periodically (consider replacing Protective Blend with Cinnamon Bark/Clove/Wild Orange blend and Soothing Blend with Helichrysum/Peppermint blend).

Precaution: Avoid Basil, Birch, Dill, Fennel, Rosemary and Wintergreen. [Also mentioned from other sources are these oils to avoid or to use with care: Camphor, Eucalyptus, Fennel, Galbanum, Hyssop, Nutmeg, Pennyroyal, Sage, Savin, Spike Lavender (not the common Lavender angustifolia), Tansy (not to be confused with Blue Tansy), Tarragon, Thuja, Thujone, Turpentine, Wormwood.]

Note: Soothing Blend has Camphor and Wintergreen. Protective Blend has Eucalyptus and Rosemary.

Other oils: Clary Sage[c], Lavender[c], Lemongrass[c] **Blends:** Joyful Blend[c], Massage Blend, Restful Blend[c]

Self confidence, *image, love*   *see* Emotional strength

Sensory Processing Disorder *(SPD)*   *see also* ADHD, Autism

Oils: Citrus oils, Lime, Wild Orange **Blends:** Grounding Blend, Joyful Blend

1-2 drops topically to the back of neck, suboccipital triangle or bottoms of feet.

Note: Many with these disorders are very sensitive to odors/touch, do not force application of oils if it is a negative experience. Apply at night on feet or some have success letting the child choose their own oils.

Other Blends: Focus Blend, Peaceful Child Blend*

*Some have had success with the blend known as Peaceful Child applied to bottoms of feet and brain/spinal reflexology points of feet after morning showering.

Sexual conditions

Aphrodisiac	*see* Aphrodisiac
Erectile dysfunction	*see* Erectile dysfunction
Fertility	*see* Infertility (female or male)
Frigidity	*see* Aphrodisiac
Impotence	*see* Libido low (female or male)
Infertility	*see* Infertility (female or male)
Libido, Low	*see* Libido low (female or male)
Sexual blocks	*see* Libido low (female or male)
Testosterone, Low	*see* Testosterone (low)

Shampoo, hair   *see* Hair care

Shigella   *see* Food poisoning

Shin splints

Oils: Lemongrass **Blends:** Soothing Blend, Soothing Blend Rub

2-4 drops Lemongrass on affected area, layer (wait 30-60 seconds for Lemongrass to penetrate) Soothing Rub over the same area. Repeat 2-4 times daily.

Other oils: Frankincense, Peppermint

Shingles

Oils: Eucalyptus[EC], Lemon[C], Marjoram, Melaleuca[C], Oregano **Blends/Products:** Basic Vitality Supplements, GI Cleansing Formula/Probiotic Defense Formula, Massage Blend

Prevention: Strengthen immune system with periodic use of the Massage Blend Technique, consistent Basic Vitality Supplements, GI Cleansing Formula/Probiotic Defense Formula cleanse (*see* Detoxification).

Help during attack: 3 drops each Eucalyptus, Lemon, Melaleuca, Oregano in capsule, 2-3x daily. Start capsules as early as the symptoms are detected. Each person is different so also consider other combinations using Frankincense, Protective Blend, Wild Orange and/or Peppermint.

Pain during an attack: Marjoram (most often mentioned), Frankincense, Geranium, Lavender or Wintergreen. Add 5ml (about 100 drops) to 4 oz spray bottle with water and spray painful areas. For sensitive skin do a skin test first.

Other oils: Clove[C], Frankincense, Geranium[EC], Lavender[C], Peppermint[E], Ravensara, Wild Orange, Wintergreen **Blends:** Protective Blend

Note: When choosing alternative oils from the list of "**Other oils:**" please review safety precautions on pages 23-28.

Shock

Oils: Grounding Blend[C], Melissa[EC], Neroli[EC], Peppermint[EC]

3-5 drops Peppermint (or Geranium, Lemon) to feet, heart area and/or back of neck to stimulate circulation.

Inhale Grounding Blend or Roman Chamomile to relax.

Other oils: Geranium[C], Helichrysum[C], Lemon[C], Melaleuca[C], Myrrh[C], Roman Chamomile[C], Ylang Ylang[C] **Blends:** Joyful Blend[C]

Shot glass

Def**inition** The shot glass (small glass associated with liquor that holds about 1-1.5 oz) is sometimes mentioned in essential oils protocols as a convenient way to add some oils or blends to a small amount of water or carrier oil. This provides

a convenient way to gargle, swish and pull or ingest the combination of oils with water or a carrier.

Siberian Fir *(Abies sibirica)*

essential oil

Properties: Analgesic, antibacterial, antifungal, anti-inflammatory, antiseptic, antispasmodic, deodorant, expectorant, mucolytic, stimulant

Addresses: Arthritis, asthma, bronchitis, cough, excess mucous, joint pain, muscle (cramps, stiffness, pain), pain killer, rheumatism, stress (tension), sinus infection, UTI

(see Safety Chart, page 23)

Sinus infection

Oils: Eucalyptus[EC], Frankincense[C], Peppermint[EC], Rosemary[EC] **Blends:** Protective Blend, Respiratory Blend[C]

Symptoms: Inhale Respiratory Blend or put 3 drops each Lemon, Lavender, Peppermint in 1/2 oz water, swish in mouth 20 sec before swallowing (consider Seasonal Blend).

Moderate infection: 2 drops each Lavender, Melaleuca or Rosemary applied with cotton swab inside nostrils or use a Neti pot.

Heavy infection: 1-4 (mild- strong) drops Eucalyptus, 2 drops each Frankincense, Rosemary, 1-2 tsp sea salt, 2 cups warm water and using Neti pot irrigate 2x or more daily.

Added help: 4 drops each Frankincense, Protective Blend, Oregano in capsule 3x daily.

Other oils: Clove[C], Elemi[C], Lemon[C], Manuka[C], Melaleuca[C], Oregano, Ravensara, Siberian Fir[C] **Blends:** Seasonal Blend

Note: When choosing alternative oils from the list of "**Other oils:**" please review safety precautions on pages 23-28.

Sjogren's syndrome   *see also* Autoimmune diseases

Oils: Frankincense[C] **Blends/Products:** Basic Vitality Supplements, Cellular Complex Blend, Soothing Blend

Consistent Basic Vitality Supplements, 8 drops or 1 capsule Cellular Complex Blend 2x daily. 2-3 drops Frankincense 2-4x daily under tongue or internally.

Symptoms: Soothing Blend for painful joints, Digestive Blend for digestive problems, Lavender or Geranium for skin problems, etc.

Other oils: Lemon[C], Melaleuca[C], Oregano[C]

Skeeter syndrome   *see also* Insect repellent, Mosquitoes

Oils: Melaleuca **Blends:** Outdoor Blend

Prevention: Apply Repellent Blend liberally without dilution to exposed areas. Typical repeat every 3-4 hours.

Reaction: 1-5 drops (depending on area) Melaleuca as soon as possible, repeat often and consistently. (*see* Shannon's SkeeterSyndrome.blogspot)

Skin blemishes

Age spots (liver spots)	*see* Age spots
Bags under eyes	*see* Bags under eyes
Cellulite reduction	*see* Cellulite reduction
Chapped skin	*see* Chapped skin
Cracked heels	*see* Cracked heels
Flabby skin	*see* Flabby skin
Itchy skin	*see* Itchy skin
Mature skin	*see* Mature skin
Moles	*see* Moles
Skin care	*see* Skin care
Skin tags	*see* Skin tags
Spider veins	*see* Spider veins
Stretch marks	*see* Stretch marks
Sunspots	*see* Sunspots
Varicose veins	*see* Varicose veins
Wrinkles	*see* Wrinkles

Skin cancer *(melanoma)*

[Basal cell carcinoma, Squamous cell carcinoma, Malignant melanoma]

Oils: Frankincense[C]

Important note: For any cancer and especially malignant melanoma seek professional medical attention immediately.

2-3 drops Frankincense area 2-3x daily. 2 drops Frankincense under tongue daily or 3 drops in capsule. Helichrysum topically to prevent scarring.

Other oils: Bergamot[C], Clove[C], Grapefruit[C], Helichrysum, Lemon[C], Lime[C], Sandalwood[C], Thyme[C]

Skin care *(primarily facial)*

Blemishes	*see* Skin Blemishes
Dry skin	*see* Chapped skin
Infants	*see* Skin care, infants
Oily skin	*see* Oily skin

Oils for basic skin care:
Cypress[EC], Geranium[EC], Jasmine[EC], Lavender[EC], Neroli[EC], Rose[EC], Arborvitae[C], Clary Sage[C], Copaiba[C], Helichrysum[C], Blue Tansy, Lemon[C], Litsea[C], Magnolia[C], Myrhh[C], Turmeric[C]

Skin care blends and products based on essential oils:
Anti-Aging Blend, Anti-Aging Moisturizer, Facial Cleanser, Foaming Face Wash, Fortifying Blend, Hydrating Cream and Facial System, Invigorating Scrub, Pore Reducing Toner, Tightening Serum, Topical Blend, Yarrow-Pomegranate Blend

Day-to-day care varies from individual to individual. Suggested protocols:

Step 1 Cleansing: Facial Cleanser or Topical Blend Foaming Face Wash (oily skin, breakout problems or men's skin).

Step 2 Toning: Invigorating Scrub or the two part, more comprehensive Facial System.

Step 3 Targeting: Essential Skin Care Tightening Serum (fine lines and wrinkles) and/or Anti-Aging Blend (trouble spots or prevention), Topical Blend (1x/week for bacterial breakouts).

Step 4 Nourishing: Anti-Aging Moisturizer (*see* Skin care) morning and night and/or Hydrating Cream for extra hydration.

essential oils
Product

Skin care products based on essential oils can be the foundation of restoring and maintaining naturally healthy skin.

BASIC NEEDS
There are available a variety of healthy basic skin care products based on quality essential oils, this includes:

Facial Cleanser: Melaleuca and Peppermint essential oils with cruciferous vegetable extracts leave skin feeling fresh and clean.

Invigorating Scrub: Grapefruit and Peppermint essential oils exfoliate while jojoba esters polish the skin. Botanicals of Mandarin Orange Extract, Jasmine Extract, and Greater Burdock Extract tone, smooth, and hydrate skin.

Pore Reducing Toner: German Chamomile, Lavender and Ylang Ylang essential oils calm sensitive skin and plant extracts increase hydration.

Tightening Serum: Frankincense, Myrrh and Hawaiian Sandalwood with other natural extracts gives hydration and firmer, younger looking skin.

Anti-Aging Moisturizer: Geranium, Frankincense, Lavender, Jasmine essential oils with unique ingredients moisturizes and improves skin tone.

Anti-Aging Blend: In a roller bottle with Frankincense, Helichrysum, Lavender, Myrrh, Rose and Sandalwood (Hawaiian) essential oils, this blend helps reduce contributing factors to the appearance of aging skin.

Hydrating Cream: Moisturizing ingredients coupled with anti-aging components designed to rejuvinate mature skin and help reduce signs of aging.

SPECIAL TREATMENTS
Detoxifying Mud Mask: The essential oils of Grapefruit, Juniper Berry and Myrrh are combined with natural earth clays, purifying minerals and nourshing botanicals for a natural clay mask. This provides purifying and detoxifying benefits while reducing the appearance of pores, fine lines and wrinkles.

Rejuvinating Process: Two step spa like treatment to give youthful glow to facial skin. Includes Lime and Wild Orange essential oils, Pumpkin enzymes, Natural Bamboo silk beads. Combines with other skin products after cleansing and before toning, targeting and nourishing.

Step 1: Apply refining polish and massage.
Step 2: Add peptide activator over polish, massage and rinse.

PROBLEM SKIN

Products formulated to address problem skin at its core.

Topical Blend: Black Cumin seed, Eucalyptus, Geranium, Ho Wood, Litsea, Melaleuca promotes a clear, smooth complexion. (see Safety Chart, page 23)

Foaming Face Wash: Eucalyptus, Geranium, Ho Wood, Litsea and Melaleuca thouroughly clease and purify skin. Licorice root extract and White Willow Bark support healthy smooth skin. A specialized blend reduces blemishes and others to sooth and calm skin.

Facial Lotion: Eucalyptus, Geranium, Ho Wood, Litsea and Melaleuca essential oils and botanical extracts improves skin texture, gives optimal hydration and a clear complexion.

EXCLUSIVE SKIN NOURISHMENT

A very high quality set of natural products for unmatched care of the skin.

Cleanser: Healthy, smooth skin with Basil, Melaleaca and Wild Orange essential oils in a natural gel that invigorates the skin while emollients nourish and hydrate.

Toner: Combines Coriander, Cypress, Palmarosa and Ylang Ylang essential oils with witch hazel, aloe and other beneficial skin care ingedients to fortify and refresh the skin and prepare the skin for the Hydrating Serum below.

Hydrating Serum: Frankincense, Helichrysum, Lavender, Myrrh, Rose and Sandalwood (Hawaiian) essential oils and specialized plant technology promotes optimal lipid balance for smoother, more youthful looking skin.

Moisturizer: Combines Geranium, Jasmine, Juniper Berry and Sea Buckthorn Berry essential oils with plant extracts for deep hydration and skin nourishment.

Legend: Preferred, Suggested, Consider

Skin care, infants

Cradle cap	*see* Cradle cap
Diaper rash	*see* Diaper rash

Skin conditions

Abscess	*see* Abscess
Acne	*see* Acne
Bruises	*see* Bruises
Calluses	*see* Calluses
Cancer	*see* Skin cancer
Cellulitis	*see* Cellulitis
Dermatitis	*see* Eczema
Ecthyma	*see* Ecthyma
Eczema	*see* Eczema
Impetigo	*see* Impetigo
Jock itch	*see* Jock itch
Parasites	*see* Parasite infections
Psoriasis	*see* Psoriasis
Rashes	*see* Rashes
Rosacea	*see* Rosacea
Scar reduction	*see* Scar reduction
Sunburn	*see* Sunburn
Vaginitis	*see* Vaginitis
Vitiligo	*see* Vitiligo

Skin conditions with weight loss

Cellulite reduction	*see* Cellulite reduction
Flabby skin	*see* Flabby skin
Stretch marks	*see* Stretch marks

Skin lesions

Boils	*see* Boils
Carbuncles	*see* Boils
Ulcerations	*see* Ulcerations, skin

Skin tags

Oils: Frankincense[C], Oregano[C] **Blends/Products:** GI Cleansing Formula/ Probiotic Defense Formula, Topical Blend

Viral based: 2-3 drops Oregano (always dilute), Topical Blend or Frankincense topically to area daily. Use GI Cleansing Formula/Probiotic Defense Formula cleanse with GI Cleansing Formula, 3 capsules daily with meals for 10 days, follow with Probiotic Defense Formula, 3 capsules daily with meals for 5 days. Rest 10 days, repeat 2x if necessary.

Skin test

Definition Applying a small amount of essential oil to a small area of skin to test for sensitivities before wider use.

Place a small amount essential oil on the inside of the elbow, underside of the forearm or underside of wrist. If there is any sensation, such as itching, warmth or stinging apply a carrier oil to relieve the feeling.

In most cases, there will be no problem with the topical applications with an oil mixed with a carrier. If there is a reaction, consider a different oil with similar benefits.

also see Safety Considerations section at front of book

Sleep apnea

Oils: Frankincense, Thyme, Ylang Ylang **Blends:** Grounding Blend, Invigorating Blend, Protective Blend, Respiratory Blend, Restful Blend

Orally: 5 drops Protective Blend, 2 Tbsp water, bedtime gargle at least 60 sec, then swish 60 sec, then spit. Internally take 1 drop of Protective Blend at bedtime.

Topical (foot): 20 drops Thyme, 5 drops each Grounding Blend, Frankincense, 30 drops FCO. Apply 2-4 drops of blend to bottoms of feet and around big toes before bedtime.

Topical (throat): 10 drops each Invigorating Blend, Frankincense, Ylang Ylang, 30 drops FCO. 4-6 drops of blend on throat and neck prior to bedtime.

Legend: Preferred, Suggested, Consider

Aromatic: Diffuse Restful Blend for restful sleep. Protective Blend or Respiratory Blend to keep sinuses clear. If you use CPAP, consider a drop in the mask.

Other oils: Lavender[C], Sandalwood **Blends:** Cleansing Blend, Soothing Blend

Sleep conditions

Insomnia	*see* Insomnia
Sleep apnea	*see* Sleep apnea
Snoring	*see* Snoring

Smell, loss of *(anosmia)*

Oils: Basil[C], Peppermint[C] **Blends:** Respiratory Blend

Clear nasal passages: Inhalation of Respiratory Blend and 2-3 drops Basil (or Melaleuca or Rosemary) to sinus areas adjacent to nose and above eyebrows. Consider possible candida and use the GI Cleansing Formula/Probiotic Defense Formula cleanse. See Detoxification and Sinus infection.

Nasal polyps: *see* Polyps

Stimulate olfactory: Consider deep inhalation of Peppermint or Respiratory Blend consistently over time. Cup & inhale 1-2x daily, 2-3 drops Basil to sinus areas adjacent to nose and above eyebrows.

Other oils: Lime, Melaleuca, Rosemary **Blends/Products:** Cellular Complex Blend, GI Cleansing Formula/Probiotic Defense Formula

Smelling salts *see* Fainting

Smoking addiction *see* Addictions

Snake bite *(supplement to antivenom serum)* *see also* Animal bites

Oils: Basil[EC], Frankincense, Helichrysum, Melaleuca **Blends:** Grounding Blend

Non-poisonous *see* Animal bites. Poisonous couple oils with immediate profession medical attention for anti-venom treatment.

Call 911 or transport. Minimize blood circulation (calm, no stimulants, limit motion). Limb lower than heart, clean and cover area. No ice, tourniquet, cutting or pain medication.

Immediately: 2-4 drops Basil/Melaleuca topically and internally. Inhale Grounding Blend or other oils to calm.

Long term: Frankincense and Helichrysum topically.

Other oils: Cinnamon Bark[E], Lavender[E], Lemon[E], Thyme[E] **Blends:** Invigorating Blend

Note: When choosing alternative oils from the list of "**Other oils:**" please review safety precautions on pages 23-28.

Snoring

Oils: Lavender, Marjoram[C], Thyme **Blends:** Protective Blend

General: Diffuse Marjoram or other relaxing oils and/or apply Lavender to bottoms of feet, back of neck, forehead, under nose and on the pillow.

Topically: 2-5 drops Thyme to bottoms of feet and big toes before retiring.

Orally: 5 drops Protective Blend, 2 Tbsp water, bedtime gargle at least 60 sec, then swish 60 sec, then spit. Internal take 1 drop Protective Blend at bedtime.

Other oils: Cypress, Eucalyptus, Marjoram, Wild Orange **Blends:** Respiratory Blend

Soaps & lotions   *see* Personal care

Soothing Blend *(help for deep tissue aches)*

essential oils
Blend

Ingredients: Blue Chamomile flower, Blue Tansy flower, Camphor bark, Helichrysum, Osmanthus flower, Peppermint, Wintergreen

Other common formulations: Clove, Helichrysum, Peppermint, Wintergreen

And: Balsam Fir, Clove, Copaiba, Helichrysum, Lemon, Peppermint, Vetiver, Wintergreen

And: Black Pepper, Hyssop, Peppermint, Spruce

Legend: Preferred, Suggested, Consider

Addresses: Arthritic pain, bruises, carpal tunnel, headaches, inflammation, joint pain, migraine, muscle pain, sprains, rheumatism

Note: For topical use only. (see Safety Chart, page 23)

Soothing Blend products

essential oils
Product

Roll-on: Gentle and quick application.

Topical Cream Rub: Soothing Blend infused in a rich, topical cream brings sensations of cooling and warmth to problem areas.

Capsules: Can be used in tandem with Blend or the Topical Cream Rub. Specific ingredients are included to provide soothing support throughout the entire body. Blend ingredients modified from the oil and rub to be safe for internal ingestion.

(see Safety Chart, page 23)

Soothing Blend for Children   see Kid's Blends

Sore nipples   see Breastfeeding

Sore throat

[also can apply to Strep throat]

Oils: Lavender[EC], Lemon[EC], Marjoram[C], Melaleuca[C], Oregano[EC] **Blends:** Protective Blend[C]

Mild: At onset 2-3 drops Lavender topically to throat every 15-20 minutes.

Strong: 2 drops each Lemon, Protective Blend in mouthful water, gargle as long as possible, swallow. Repeat every 1-2 hours until pain subsides. Then 2-3 times daily for at least two days.

Extra strong: Add 1-2 drops Oregano (hot, always dilute) or other oil from above.

Children: Mild or Strong oils combinations recommended above applied topically on throat, around ears and on bottoms of feet. At least 3-4x daily for 2-3 days.

If heavy soreness has developed: Use above plus 1 drop each Lemon and Oregano with 10 drops FCO, do lymphatic massage on neck and follow with warm compress.

Laryngitis: Oregano (hot, always dilute) and Marjoram or Frankincense as a gargle.

Other oils: Cypress^{EC}, Eucalyptus^{EC}, Frankincense, Geranium^{EC}, Manuka^C, Sandalwood^C, Siberian Fir^C, Thyme^{EC}

Sores, open	*see* Ulcerations, skin

Sorrow	*see* Grief

Spasmodic cough	*see* Cough

Spasms *(abnormal muscle contraction)*	*see* Muscle cramps

SPD	*see* Sensory Processing Disorder

Spearmint *(Mentha spicata)*

essential oil

Properties: Antiseptic, appetite stimulant, digestive, expectorant, insecticide, stimulant

Addresses: ADHD, asthma, bronchitis, candida, child birth (eases labor), cystitis, dry skin, eczema, flatulence, gums (sore), headaches, hepatitis, kidney stones, menstrual problems (heavy periods), muscle pain, nausea, nerve pain, sinusitis, stomach spasms, tooth problems, ulcers, vaginitis

(see Safety Chart, page 23)

Spider bites

Oils: Basil^C **Blends:** Cleansing Blend^C

Dab Basil (or other recommended oils) topically directly on bite, repeat every 1-2 hours. With children or sensitive skin dilute with a carrier oil.

Precaution: With any suspicion of black widow, brown recluse, etc. seek professional medical attention.

Other oils: Peppermint **Blends:** Outdoor Blend

Spider veins
see Varicose veins

Spikenard *(Nardostachys jatamansi)*

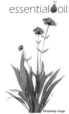
essential oil

Properties: Antibacterial, antifungal, anti-inflammatory, antispasmodic, calming, deodorant, sedative

Addresses: Agitation, allergies, anxiety, body odor, candidiasis, cellulitis, conjunctivitis, depression, emotional fatigue, flatulence, fungal infections, hemorrhoids, hormonal balance, indigestion, insomnia, mature skin, menstrual conditions, migraine, muscle cramps, PMS, nausea, rashes, staph infections, stress, ulcers

(see Safety Chart, page 23)

Spina bifida
see Back conditions

Spinal conditions
see Back conditions

Spinal stenosis
see Back conditions

Splinters
see also Cuts and wounds

Oils: Frankincense^{EC}, Lavender^{EC}, Melaleuca^{EC} **Blends:** Cleansing Blend^C, Protective Blend^C

Follow these basic steps:

Disinfect: 1-2 drop Protective Blend topically on area.

Remove exposed: Use fingernails, tweezers or sfy tape.

Remove unexposed: Disinfect tweezers and needle and attempt, if not easily removed, apply 1-3 drops Cleansing Blend on splinter at bedtime, cover, should come out or be easily removed in morning.

Antibiotic: Topical apply Lavender, Frankincense, Myrrh or Protective Blend every 4-6 hours.

Calming: If a child, rub palms together with 2-3 drops of Lavender and let child inhale.

Other oils: Copaiba^C, Lemon^C, Myrrh^{EC}

Sprains

Blend for pain, circulation and to encourage repair: Massage Blend

Pain: Soothing Blend^c, Lavender^{EC}

Circulation, inflammation and warming: Clove^c, Cypress

Encourage tissue repair: Helichrysum^c (nerve), Lemongrass^c (ligaments, tendons), Marjoram^c (muscle)

First 24-48 hours: For pain 1-5 drops Lavender or Marjoram and also Soothing Blend if pain intense apply topically immediately and often. Combine with RICE treatment (Rest, Ice, Compress, Elevate).

After 24-48 hours (when swelling is controlled**):** Use a blend of oils to limit pain, increase circulation and encourage tissue repair. Massage Blend or Soothing Blend combined with Cypress, Helichrysum, Lemongrass and Marjoram are highly recommended. Apply with hot/cold compresses or hot/cold foot-baths (if an ankle). Compress or bath should include the blend of oils mentioned and hot/cold should be alternated every 5-10 minutes for 3-4 rotations. Repeat every 3-12 hours depending on severity.

Special Precautions: If after 2-4 days sprain is not better there may be a broken bone or severely torn ligament, seek professional medical help.

Other oils:

Pain: Birch, White Fir^c, Wintergreen **Blends:** Tension Blend

Circulation, inflammation and warming: Cinnamon Bark, Eucalyptus^{EC}, Ginger^c, Oregano, Peppermint, Roman Chamomile^c, Rosemary^c

Encourage tissue repair: Frankincense

Spray bottle

 Definition

A convenient way to apply oils to a large or sensitive area. Mixing oils with water in a spray bottle is called a Spritz. Other times the recommendation may be to mix oils or blends with a carrier oil. It is best then to use a glass bottle. Small glass bottles with spray tops are available commercially as well as spray tops that can be put directly on the common 15ml essential oil bottles.

Spritz

Definition Adding an essential oil to a bottle of water with a spray top to apply a fine mist of oil and water. Convenient for applying oils to large or sensitive areas. Shake thoroughly before spraying.

Spurs
see Bone spurs

Squamous cell carcinoma
see Skin cancer

Stamina complex
see Energy & Stamina complex

Staph infections
see also MRSA

Oils: Frankincense[C], Oregano[C] **Blends:** Protective Blend[C]

4 drops each Protective Blend and Oregano in capsule 2-3x daily or 4 drops each of Oregano and Melaleuca and/or 1 drop Frankincense in capsule 2-3x daily.

Open sore: 2-4 drops Frankincense topically to area or other oils with a carrier.

Other oils: Cinnamon Bark[C], Clove[C], Eucalyptus[C], Lemon[C], Lemongrass[C], Melaleuca[C], Spikenard[C], Thyme[C] **Blends:** Anti-Aging Blend[C]

Note: When choosing alternative oils from the list of "**Other oils:**" please review safety precautions on pages 23-28.

Staphylococcus aureus
see Food poisoning

Star Anise *(Illicium verum)*

essential oil

Properties: Analgesic, antibacterial, antifungal, antioxidant, antiseptic, antispasmodic, aphrodisiac, calming, digestive, disinfectant, diuretic, expectorant, laxative, sedative, stimulant (digestive)

Addresses: Arthritis, cough, digestive problems, muscle cramps, insomnia, low libido (men)

Caution: Extra cautions are noted for this oil in Safety Chart. (see Safety Chart, page 23)

Steadying Blend *(a Yoga blend)*

Blend

Ingredients: Lavender, Cedarwood, Frankincense, Cinnamon Bark, Sandalwood, Black Pepper, Patchouli

Addresses: Brings a firm trust in self, so life can be approached with calm strength.

(see Safety Chart, page 23)

Steam tent

Definition Add an essential oil or blend to steaming hot bowl of water. Place towel over head, drape around bowl and breathe in vapors.

Stings   *see* Insect bites

Stomachache

Oils: Fennel^E, Ginger^C, Peppermint^EC **Blends:** Digestive Blend^C

2-5 drops Digestive Blend supplemented with 1-3 drops of Coriander or if Digestive Blend not available consider Coriander, Fennel, Ginger and/or Peppermint neat on abdomen or in capsule.

Children and sensitive skin: Add 4-10 drops carrier oil topically to tummy.

Infants: Rub on bottoms of feet.

Other oils: Basil^C, Cinnamon Bark^E, Clove^C, Coriander^C, Cumin^C, Cypress^C, Green Mandarin^EC, Litsea^C, Marjoram^EC, Myrrh^C, Pink Pepper^C, Roman Chamomile^EC, Rosemary^EC, Spearmint^C, Star Anise^C, Tangerine^C, Wild Orange^C

Note: When choosing alternative oils from the list of "**Other oils:**" please review safety precautions on pages 23-28.

Stomach cramps   *see* Stomachache

Stomach flu *(viral gastroenteritis)*   *see also* Flu

Pain/discomfort: Digestive Blend; Antiviral: Frankincense^C, Oregano^C, Thyme

4 drops each Digestive Blend and Frankincense in capsule 2-3x daily.

Additional for Pain/discomfort: 3-4 drops Digestive Blend topically to abdomen. Also consider Ginger or Peppermint (with carrier).

Children and infants: Children dilute with carrier and apply to tummy, babies dilute with carrier and apply to bottoms of the feet.

Alternative for viral infection (adults): 4 drops each Oregano, Thyme, fill with FCO in capsule, 2-3x daily.

Other oils: Pain/discomfort: Fennel, Ginger, Peppermint, Sandalwood, Yarrow^C

Antiviral: Cinnamon Bark^C, Clove^C, Eucalyptus^C, Helichrysum^C, Lemon^C, Melaleuca^C, Melissa^C, Myrrh^C, Protective Blend^C

Note: When choosing alternative oils from the list of "**Other oils:**" please review safety precautions on pages 23-28.

Stomatitis *(mouth sores)*

see Canker sores and Cold sores for these health concerns.

Oils: Clove, Frankincense, Lavender, Oregano **Blends:** Protective Blend^C

4 drops Protective Blend to 2 Tbsp FCO, use oil pulling for 5-10 minutes 2-3x daily.

Pain/open sores: 2-4 drops each Frankincense, Lavender in 1 Tbsp FCO, use oil pulling with mixture as needed.

Other oils: Bergamot^E, Geranium^E, Melaleuca, Myrrh

Strep throat   *see* Sore throat

Stress

Oils: Clary Sage^{EC}, Frankincense^C, Geranium^{EC}, Lavender^{EC}, Wild Orange^C, Ylang Ylang^C **Blends:** Grounding Blend^C, Invigorating Blend, Joyful Blend^C, Massage Blend, Reassuring Blend, Restful Blend^C

There are numerous oils many have had positive experiences with for stress. Oils affect each person differently, experiment to see which gives the most effective help. It is suggested you try the blends and/or the Preferred oils first.

Home: Topically to temples, behind ears o other stress points. 3-4 drops in warm bath, Massage Blend Technique, foot or hand massage.

Home/office: Diffuse.

On the go: Make an inhaler or roller ball dispenser, cup & inhale.

Other oils: Basil[C], Bergamot[C], Blue Tansy[C], Cardamom[C], Cypress[C], Elemi[C], Grapefruit[C], Jasmine[C], Lemon[C], Lime[C], Magnolia[C], Manuka[C], Marjoram[C], Neroli[C], Patchouli[C], Petitgrain[C], Roman Chamomile[C], Rose[C], Sandalwood[C], Siberian Fir[C], Spikenard[C], Tangerine[C], Turmeric[C], Vetiver[EC] **Blends:** Comforting Blend, Tension Blend, Uplifting Blend

Stretch marks

Oils: Frankincense, Geranium, Helichrysum[E], Lavender[C] **Blends/ Products:** Anti-Aging Moisturizer (*see* Skin care)

Anti-aging Moisturizer (containing Lavender, Jasmine, Geranium, and Frankincense) augmented with Grapefruit oil. Apply topically to area 2-3x daily.

Or 1 oz VCO with 12 drops each Lavender, Frankincense, Geranium and Helichrysum. Apply topically to area 2-3x daily.

Other oils: Copaiba[C], Cypress[C], Grapefruit[C], Green Mandarin[EC], Myrrh[C], Neroli[EC], Tangerine[C], Rosemary

Stroke

Oils: Frankincense[C], Melissa[C] **Blends:** Grounding Blend[C], Massage Blend[C]

ATTENTION: Seek immediate professional medical attention with any symptoms of a stroke.

After stroke help: Massage 1-2 drops Massage Blend over heart and 1-2 drops of Frankincense under tongue 2-5x daily.

Couple with the Massage Blend Technique daily (or more often) and add Frankincense to inflammation phase (step 3). Consistently use Basic Vitality Supplements.

After stroke help for hemorrhagic stroke: Consider lightly massaging 1-2 drops Melissa on head as close as possible to stroke area.

Other oils: Basil[C], Copaiba[C], Cypress[C], Grapefruit[C], Lavender[C], Peppermint

Stuffy nose   *see* Allergies or Colds

Sty

Oils: Lavender, Melaleuca **Blends:** Protective Blend[C]

Older children/adults: Topically dab one of these oils with finger tip around eye socket or rub on palms of hands, cup hand over eye, nose and mouth and hold for 1-2 minutes while your own breath carries oils to the eye.

Younger children: Use hard shell eye patch (pharmacy) with 2 drops of oils on 1/3 of a cotton pad placed in patch with oils side of cotton away from eye. Place over affected eye. Also apply oils on reflexology points.

Note: Essential oils must not be used directly in the eye. They will not injure the eye but there will be very uncomfortable stinging. If this happens do not flush the eye with water, rather use FCO or olive oil.

Caution children not to rub eyes and with small children when oils are put on feet, place socks on feet so oils are not accidentally transferred to eyes.

Other oils: Frankincense, Helichrysum

Suboccipital triangle

Definition An application point for essential oils recommended for arterial flow to the brain and key neurological tissue. Place the fingers on the suboccipital protuberance (little bump at top of the spine on the back of the neck) then just below this grip the large muscle tissue and roll the fingers off to the side. This depression just behind and below the ear is the suboccipital triangle.

Sudorific *(promotes sweating)*

This is a partial list of some oils with sudorific properties.

Oils: Lavender^C, Roman Chamomile^C, Rosemary^C, Thyme^C

Suicide threat   *see* Depression

Sunburn   *see also* Sunscreen

Oils: Frankincense, Lavender^C, Melaleuca^C, Peppermint

20 drops each Lavender, Peppermint to 2 oz spray bottle. Fill with water or FCO. Shake and apply to area every 2 hours, repeat 4-6 times. Continue with 20 drops each Lavender, Frankincense with 1 oz water 2-4x daily. If blistering add 20 drops Melaleuca.

Other oils: Black Pepper, Blue Tansy^E, Cellular Complex Blend, Geraniuim, Helichrysum^C, Roman Chamomile^C, Sandalwood^C

Sunscreen   *see also* Sunburn

Oils: Helichrysum^C, Lavender^C, Sandalwood^C

60 drops each Helichrysum, Sandalwood (or Lavender) to 2 oz spray bottle. Fill with FCO. This is a moderate sunscreen and may be sprayed on and used as any commercial sunscreen.

Before and after lotion: 8-10 drops each Helichrysum, Lavender and Sandalwood with 5 oz Hand & Body Lotion, 1.5 oz filtered water in 8 oz squeeze bottle. Shake and use before and after sun exposure.

Sunspots

Oils: Clove^C, Lemongrass^C **Blends:** Topical Blend^C

Fungus (tinea versicolor): Use topical application of Topical Blend or other antifungal oils (Clove, Eucalyptus, Lemongrass, Melaleuca). May require weeks of consistent application.

Excessive sun exposure: *see* Age spots

Other oils: Eucalyptus, Melaleuca, Oregano^C, Rosemary^C, Thyme^C
Blends: Protective Blend^C

Legend: Preferred, Suggested, Consider

Sunstroke
see Heat exhaustion

Superficial phlebitis
see Blood clots

Supplements

essential oils
Product

A number of essential oil based and related supplements are offered by many sources to help supplement nutritional needs. Following are some found in this book:

Children	*see* Children's supplements
Energy & Stamina	*see* Energy & Stamina Complex
Fruits & Vegetables	*see* Fruit & Vegetable mix
Nutritional	*see* Basic Vitality supplements
Probiotics	*see* Probiotic Defense formula
Vegan	*see* Vegan products

Surface cleaning
see Household care

Surgery

Oils: Basil, Clary Sage, Cypress, Frankincense, Lemon, Oregano, Vetiver
Blends/Products: GI Cleansing Formula/Probiotic Defense Formula, Grounding Blend, Massage Blend, Protective Blend

Pre-Op:

Two weeks prior: Daily drink lots of water with 2 drops Lemon, use the Massage Blend Technique at least 2x weekly or more.

One week prior: 2-4 drops Protective Blend on bottoms of feet daily.

Two days prior: 2-3 drops each Grounding Blend, Frankincense and Vetiver with massage to shoulders, neck and brain stem. 1-2 drops each Basil, Clary Sage, Frankincense, Protective Blend to region of surgery.

Post-Op (as soon as possible consider the following):

Increase circulation and additional help: Basil and Cypress to topically area of surgery (skin test oils first).

Excess bleeding: Geranium and Helichrysum topically.

Muscle cramps: Topically apply Massage Blend or Clary Sage with Birch (skin test) together.

Inflammation and MRSA: Protective Blend and Oregano (skin test) with carrier topically. Diffuse Frankincense and Protective Blend in room 2-3x daily or use spritz with 2-3 drops each oil and water, spray bed and area.

Intestinal flora: Consider GI Cleansing Formula/Probiotic Defense Formula cleanse to re-establish intestinal flora. *see* Detoxification.

Stress and balance: Diffuse Grounding Blend, Lavender or other soothing oil, with Massage Blend Technique as soon as possible, 2x weekly minimum.

Other oils: Geranium, Helichrysum, Peppermint

Susquiterpenes   *see* Chemical constituents

Swallowing difficulty   *see also* Heartburn
[Achalasia, Dysphagia, Esophagitis Odynophagia]

Oils: Frankincense[c], Helichrysum

Frankincense or blend of 2 drops each Basil, Frankincense, Myrrh, 1-2 drops Cinnamon Bark to taste. Add to small amount of water and using a straw let it 'trickle' down throat to maximize soothing esophagus. Repeat at least daily.

Added help: Same blend topically on throat and chest area.

Achalasia: Add 2 drops Helichrysum to blend.

Other oils: Basil, Cinnamon Bark, Myrrh

Swelling   *see* Edema

Swine flu   *see* Flu

Swollen ankles   *see* Edema

Legend: Preferred, Suggested, Consider

Tachycardia
see Heart conditions

Tangerine *(Citrus reticulata)*

Properties: Anticoagulent, antidepressant, anti-inflammatory, calming, digestive, laxative, sedative

Addresses: Anxiety, calming, cellulite reduction, children's stomachaches, constipation, depression, diarrhea, digestive cramps, edema, flatulence, grief, hiccups, insomnia, irritability, liver conditions, muscle pain, obesity, parasite infections, sadness, stress, stretch marks, stomachache

(see Safety Chart, page 23)

Tansy
see Blue Tansy

Tape worms
see Parasite infections

Tea Tree
see **Melaleuca**

Tee shirt tent

A technique to facilitate deeply inhaling oils. Layer the desired oils on your chest and lightly rub in. Put on a tee shirt. Let the oils sit on your skin, while you cup and inhale from your hands deeply for several minutes. Then pull the neck of your tee shirt up over your mouth and nose and breathe in deeply for several minutes until the aroma begins to dissipate. If you feel like you are not getting enough oxygen, take a break for a couple breaths, then resume. As you do this, you will feel the oils begin to penetrate deeper and deeper into the lungs and will even feel a cooling sensation in your lungs.

Teeth care
see Oral hygiene

Teeth conditions

Grinding teeth	*see* Teeth grinding
Gum conditions	*see* Gum conditions
Teething	*see* Teething
Tooth abscess	*see* Abscess

[Abscess, Cavities, Toothache]

Oils: Clove[C] **Blends/Products:** Protective Blend[C], Protective Blend Toothpaste

Pain: 1-2 drops each Clove and Protective Blend to area as needed (dilute for children).

Hygiene during time of painful conditions: Along with regular brushing/ flossing using Protective Blend Toothpaste use an Oil Pulling technique 2-3 times a day. Add 2-5 drops Protective Blend and 1-3 drops of Clove to a mouthful of warm water. Oil Pull this mixture for 5-10 minutes in mouth. Do not swallow mixture when finished. Add Lemon or Peppermint to improve taste. Continue regular oral hygiene, see dentist.

Adults: Clove can be rubbed directly on painful tooth/gum area for immediate relief.

Children: Dilute Clove with pleasant tasting carrier before applying.

Special Precautions: Clove is a "hot" oil and can be uncomfortable for some, so consider using it diluted with a carrier oil.

Other oils: Lemon, Myrrh[EC], Oregano, Peppermint

Teeth grinding

Oils: Lavender[C] **Blends:** Restful Blend[C]

To improve restful sleep, diffuse Restful Blend or Lavender at bedtime or 1-2 drops of Restful Blend or Lavender on forehead at bedtime. For children also massage Lavender or Restful Blend on bottoms of feet.

Other oils: Marjoram **Blends:** Basic Vitality Supplements, Massage Blend, Soothing Blend

Teething

Oils: Clove, Lavender[C], Roman Chamomile[EC]

Legend: Preferred, Suggested, Consider

Three techniques:

Touch open top of bottle (partial drop of oil) and rub on gums.

1 drop oil and 3-4 drops FCO and rub directly on the gums.

1 drop oil and 3-4 drops FCO and rub on outside of jaw line.

Other oils: Myrrh

Temperature   see Fever

Temporomandibular joint syndrome   see TMJ

Tendinitis (Tendonitis)

Oils: Birch, Cypress, Lemongrass[C], Peppermint[C] **Blends:** Massage Blend[C], Soothing Blend[C]

2-3 drops Soothing Blend or Birch to affected area for pain and inflammation, follow with 2-3 drops Lemongrass to encourage tissue repair. Layer with Peppermint to "drive" oils deeper or use a warm compress. Repeat 2-3x daily. Cypress provides additional help.

Other oils: Basil, Helichrysum[EC], Lavender[C], Lemon[C], Oregano[C], Wintergreen[C]

Tennis elbow   see Tendinitis

Tension Blend (for headaches and other tense aches)

(comes in roll-on)

essential oils
Blend

Ingredients: Basil, Cilantro, Frankincense, Lavender, Marjoram, Peppermint, Roman Chamomile, Rosemary, Wintergreen

Another common formulation: Basil, Helichrysum, Lavender, Marjoram, Peppermint, Roman Chamomile

Addresses: Headaches, stress, tension

(see Safety Chart, page 23)

Terpenes   see Chemical constituents

Testicular cancer
see Cancer

Testosterone (low)

Oils: Clary Sage, Geranium, Sandalwood **Blends:** Basic Vitality Supplements

1-2 drops Sandalwood (Clary Sage or Geranium) with 1 Tbsp FCO, apply topically to testicles and bottoms of feet. Diffuse or cup & inhale. Consistent Basic Vitality Supplements.

If caused by infection, GI Cleansing Formula cleanse. *See* Detoxification.

Other oils: Rosemary **Blends/Products:** GI Cleansing Formula, Grounding Blend

Throat conditions
see Nose/throat conditions

Thrombosis
see Blood clots

Thrush (oral candidiasis)
see also Candidiasis

Oils: Clove, Oregano **Blends:** GI Cleansing Formula/Probiotic Defense Formula, Protective Blend

Children: 2 drops Protective Blend and/or 1 drop Oregano to bottoms of feet. For an infant premix oils, apply 1 drop of blend. Cover with socks to avoid accidental transfer. Continue 3-5 days. If symptoms continue consider Candida. If child is breastfed consider Candida cleanse for mother.

Adults: GI Cleansing Formula/Probiotic Defense Formula protocol, 1-3 GI Cleansing Formula capsules daily with meals for 10 days. Follow with Probiotic Defense Formula for 5 days. Simultaneously gargle 3-4x daily water and 1 drop each of Protective Blend and Clove, continue 2 days after symptoms subside.

Other oils: Lavender[C], Melaleuca[C], Thyme[C]

Legend: Preferred, Suggested, Consider

Thyme, ct thymol *(Thymus vulgaris)*

essential oil

Properties: Antibacterial, antibiotic, antifungal, antioxidant, antiseptic, antispasmodic, astringent, disinfectant

Addresses: Asthma, bronchitis, cold and flu, constipation, cough, cuts and wounds, dermatitis, insomnia, skin disorders, sore throat, stomachache, throat infections, yeast infection

(see Safety Chart, page 23)

Thyroid conditions

Goiter	*see* Goiter
Graves' disease	*see* Hyperthyroidism
Hashimoto's disease	*see* Hypothyroidism
Hyperthyroidism	*see* Hyperthyroidism
Hypothyroidism	*see* Hypothyroidism
Thyroid nodules	*see* Thyroid nodules

Thyroid nodules

Oils: Frankincense, Grapefruit[C], Lemon[C], Sandalwood **Blends:** Basic Vitality Supplements, GI Cleansing Formula/Probiotic Defense Formula

GI Cleansing Formula/Probiotic Defense Formula detoxification, Basic Vitality Supplements, 2-4 drops Sandalwood 1:1 with EVCO topically to thyroid area 2-3x daily. Additional help rotate Sandalwood with Frankincense every day plus the Massage Blend Technique periodically.

For symptoms:

Pain: Soothing Blend Rub

Tiredness and depression: Citrus oils, Joyful Blend or Peppermint

Anxiety and irritability: Grounding Blend and Melissa

Other oils: Geranium, Lemongrass, Myrrh **Blends:** Massage Blend, Grounding Blend

Ticks   *see also* Lyme disease

Oils: Basil, Lemon, Cinnamon Bark, Lavender, Lemongrass, Melaleuca, Thyme, Cleansing Blend

Avoid ticks: Outdoor Blend or if in an area of high tick concentration use strong oils such as Basil, Cinnamon Bark or Thyme with carrier as an additional repellent.

Tick attached to skin: To remove some recommend tweezers or a tick removal tool. Grasp tick near its head (not stomach area) and gently remove upward. Others suggest putting a drop or two of essential oil like Melaleuca or other strong oils to "encourage" tick to loosen hold on skin and then remove with tweezers. Save tick in ziplock in freezer in event there are complications.

After removal: Apply antibacterial oils such as Melaleuca or Cleansing Blend. If there is a follow on rash, headache, fever or flu-like symptoms see a doctor.

Tighten skin   *see* Personal care and Skin care

Tinnitus *(ringing in ears)*

Oils: Basil, Frankincense, Helichrysum[C]

Protocol 1: 1 drop each Frankincense, Basil and apply to back of ear and down jaw line to chin on each ear. Repeat starting at top of ear and down front of ear and jaw line. Repeat every 1-4 hours.

Protocol 2: Blend 4 drops each Cypress, Helichrysum, Lavender, Rosemary, let stand 24 hours, add 1 oz FCO. Put 5-7 drops of blend in palm and apply with fingers starting at front of ear, around outside rim of ear and down to lobe. Continue in depression behind and below ear and down jaw line. Repeat until oil in palm is used. Let recipient breathe in palm. Repeat 2-3 times daily.

Also consider: 2 drops Helichrysum in 1/2 a cotton ball inserted into ear. Some report a root cause may be Candida and using GI Cleansing Formula/Probiotic Defense Formula cleanse is a help.

Other oils: Geranium, Peppermint **Blends/Products:** GI Cleansing Formula/Probiotic Defense Formula

Legend: Preferred, Suggested, Consider

Tissue cup

 Definition A technique for using oils that may need to be inhaled periodically during the day. Using a small disposable container such as the Glad Mini Round cup (4 oz, BPA free). Put a tissue in the cup and add a few drops of the desired oil then seal with the provided cap. During the day the cap may be removed and the oil inhaled then resealed for later use.

TMJ *(temporomandibular joint syndrome)*

Oils: Frankincense[C] **Blends:** Anti-Aging Blend, Soothing Blend[C]

Soothing Blend Rub or 2-3 drops Frankincense or Anti-Aging Blend on TMJ just below the ear and around to back of neck. Repeat 2-3x daily.

Other blends: Tension Blend, White Fir

Tobacco   *see* Addictions

Toenail fungus   *see* Nail fungus

Toenails, strengthen   *see* Nails, strengthen

Tonsillitis

Oils: Oregano **Blends:** Protective Blend

Older children: 2-3 drops Protective Blend to mouthful of water and gargle for as long as possible, then swallow (some prefer to spit out). Repeat every 1-2 hours. (Oregano is also effective but difficult to use without careful dilution or may be applied to bottoms of feet).

Younger children: 2-3 drops Protective Blend to spoonful of applesauce, swallow. Repeat every 1-2 hours.

Youngest children: 2-3 drops Protective Blend with 4-6 drops FCO, apply topically to throat area every 1-2 hours.

Other oils: Clove[C], Ginger[EC], Lavender[C], Lemon[EC], Melaleuca[C]

Topical Blend *(clear skin blemishes)*

Blend

Ingredients: Black Cumin seed, Eucalyptus, Geranium, Ho Wood, Litsea, Melaleuca

Addresses: Acne, athlete's foot, facial blemishes, itchy scalp, infected nails, toe nail fungus, skin lesions

(see Safety Chart, page 23)

Topical Blend products

essential oils
Product

Roll-on: Gentle and quick application.

Facial lotion: Non-greasy moisturizer provides hydration and improves skin texture

Foaming face wash: Cleanses skin and promotes cell renewal and clear, smooth complexion.

(see Safety Chart, page 23)

Tourette syndrome

Oils: Frankincense, Invigorating Blend, Vetiver **Blends:** Focus Blend, Grounding Blend^c, Peaceful Child Blend, Restful Blend

Calm/improve concentration: 2-5 drops Grounding Blend, Restful Blend or Invigorating Blend with 1-2 drops Frankincense or Vetiver. Application can be done in a number of ways:

Topically on bottoms of feet and back of neck morning, midday and late afternoon.

Carry an inhaler, direct inhalation, terracotta pendant for children.

Diffuse if surrounding environment allows.

Focus Blend is blend in roller bottle for helping maintain focus, can be carried or applied to a pendant and used anytime.

Relaxed sleep: 2-3 drops Frankincense, Lavender and Restful Blend topically to feet, under nose, on pillow case or diffuse at night.

Other helpful hints:

Some children with neurological problems are sensitive to smell and may resist use of oils. Do not force but apply to feet after asleep.

Legend: Preferred, Suggested, Consider

Experiment with various oils to find the best alternatives.

Rotate oils on weekly or monthly basis to get maximum benefits.

2 drops Frankincense under tongue daily.

Note: Some have had success with the blend known as Peaceful Child applied to bottoms of feet and brain/spinal reflexology points of feet after morning shower.

Other oils: Clary Sage, Helichrysum, Lavender, Lemon, Marjoram, Myrrh, Ylang Ylang

Toxemia   *see* Pregnancy

Travel help

Many suggest carrying the Basic 10 Oils Kit while traveling to provide basic protection and responsiveness to emergency situations.

Air travel with oils	*see* Air travel with oils
Jet lag	*see* Jet lag
Motion sickness	*see* Motion sickness
Traveler's diarrhea	*see* Diarrhea

Traveler's diarrhea   *see* Diarrhea

Tremors   *see* Essential tremors

Trigeminal neuralgia   *see* Neuralgia

Tuberculosis

Oils: Frankincense[C], Oregano[EC], Peppermint[EC] **Blends:** Protective Blend[C]

Diffuse, cup & inhale and/or apply topically to back, chest and bottoms of feet some of the referenced oils such as below.

Not many protocols are referenced in the literature but an experienced essential oils user, with no direct experience with TB, but some study of the nature of the disease, suggested a blend of 6 parts Protective Blend, 3 parts Oregano, 1 part Frankincense taken in capsule 2x daily.

Other oils: Cinnamon Bark, Eucalyptus[EC], Lemon[EC], Lemongrass,

Melaleuca, Sandalwood[EC], Thyme[EC]

Note: When choosing alternative oils from the list of "**Other oils:**" please review safety precautions on pages 23-28.

Turmeric *(Curcuma longa)*

essential oil

Properties: Antibacterial, antibiotic, antidepressant, antifungal, anti-inflammatory, antimicrobial, antioxidant, antiparasitic, antiseptic, antitumoral, calming, diuretic

Addresses: Allergies, arthritis, fungal infections, joint pain and stiffness, liver support, muscle pain, skin blemishes, stress

Some mention Turmeric has been used to help Alzheimer's, mental confusion, dementia, epilepsy and memory loss as well as interesting research reports relative to Turmeric and various types of cancer.

(see Safety Chart, page 23)

Tumors

Abscess	*see* Abscess
Cancerous	*see* Cancer
Cyst	*see* Cyst
Lipoma	*see* Lipoma
Polyp	*see* Polyps
Thyroid nodules	*see* Thyroid nodules
Uterine fibroids	*see* Uterine fibroids

Benign tumors in general:

Oils: Frankincense **Blends:** Cellular Complex Blend

2-3 drops Frankincense and/or Cellular Complex Blend topically to area of tumor 2-3x daily. If internal, oils under tongue, rub on bottoms of feet or in capsule.

Other oils: Basil, Bergamot[E], Copaiba[C], Cypress, Eucalyptus, Lavender, Lemongrass, Marjoram, Oregano, Peppermint, Roman Chamomile[E], Thyme

U - V

Ulcerations, skin (open sores)

Oils: Frankincense^EC, Lavender^EC, Helichrysum^C

Simple: 2-3 drops Lavender topically to area.

Serious: Blend Frankincense and Helichrysum, apply 2-4 drops at least 2x daily, consistency is important.

Consider: Root cause may be candida or other internal problems. *See* Detoxification.

Other oils: Cypress^C, Geranium^EC, Manuka^C, Myrrh^EC **Blends:** Topical Blend^C

Ulcerative colitis   see Inflammatory bowel disease

Ulcers (peptic ulcer, H. pylori)   see also Diabetes (diabetic ulcers)
[Ulcers stomach (gastric ulcer), Ulcers intestines (duodenal ulcer)]

Oils: Frankincense^C, Lemongrass, Peppermint^C **Blends:** Digestive Blend

Immediate relief: 2-4 drops Peppermint to 1/4 cup water or juice and drink (may be "hot" to some).

Long term help: 4 drops each Digestive Blend, Frankincense and Lemongrass in capsule, take 2x daily.

Children: Rub above blend with carrier oil on tummy 2x daily.

Other oils: Basil^C, Geranium^EC, Lemon^EC, Roman Chamomile^C

Ulcers, venous   see Varicose veins

Ulcerative colitis   see Inflammatory bowel disease

Umbilical hernia   see Hernia

Underarm odor   see Body odor

Uplifting Blend

essential oils
Blend (comes in a roll-on dispenser)

Ingredients: Cinnamon Bark, Clove, Ginger, Lemon Myrtle, Nutmeg, Star Anise, Vanilla, Wild Orange, Zdravetz

Addresses: An emotional health blend to uplift the spirit and cheer the soul.

(see Safety Chart, page 23)

Upset stomach   see Stomachache

Urethra infection   see UTI

Urination difficulty, male   see Prostate conditions

Urination, painful   see Prostate conditions or UTI

Uterine cancer   see Cancer

Uterine fibroids

Oils: Frankincense[C], Sandalwood

Prevention/reduction: 2-3 drops Frankincense under tongue morning and night. GI Cleansing Formula/Probiotic Defense Formula cleanse. *See* Candidiasis.

Pain/cramps: 8-12 drops Sandalwood in capsule at onset, second day reduce to 6-8 drops. Or 2-4 drops each Cypress and Rosemary topically to abdomen, follow with warm compress.

Excessive Bleeding: 6-8 drops Frankincense internally vaginally on the end of a tampon or in capsule with FCO inserted upon retiring.

Other oils: Cypress, Eucalyptus, Geranium, Rosemary **Blends/Products:** GI Cleansing Formula/Probiotic Defense Formula

UTI *(urinary tract infection)*   *see also* Bladder wall inflammation

[Bladder infection (cystitis), Bladder wall inflammation (interstitial cystitis), Kidney infection, Urethra infection (urethritis)]

Oils: Frankincense, Lemon[EC], Oregano[C] **Blends:** Protective Blend

Adults: 2 drops Frankincense, 6 drops Protective Blend, 6 drops Oregano in capsule 3x daily. 1/2 cup unsweetened cranberry juice 3x daily.
Children: 3 drops Protective Blend in 1/2 cup of unsweetened cranberry juice sweetened with honey, 3x daily. Topically 1-2 drops Oregano with 2+ drops carrier oil to bottoms of feet 3x daily.

Everyone: Also rub Cypress topically on lower abdomen 2x daily. Continue oils one week after symptoms subside. Drink lots of water, add 1-2 drops of Lemon to each glass of water.

Other oils: Cassia, Cinnamon Bark, Clove, Cypress^C, Juniper Berry^EC, Lemongrass^C, Melaleuca^C, Sandalwood^EC, Siberian Fir^C, Thyme^EC

Note: When choosing alternative oils from the list of "**Other oils:**" please review safety precautions on pages 23-28.

Uveitis (iritis)
see Eyesight failing

Vaginitis

[leukorrhea]

Oils: Frankincense, Lavender^C, Melaleuca^EC

Yeast (fungal) infection: see protocols under Candida, Lavender topically to soothe discomfort.

Bacterial infection: 2-5 drops each Lavender, Melaleuca, 1 Tbsp EVCO, soak tampon. Use nightly for a full week.

Leukorrhea: If light this may be normal but if unusual this vaginal discharge may be from a vaginal infection or estrogen imbalance.

Other oils: Bergamot^E, Cinnamon Bark^C, Eucalyptus^C, Roman Chamomile^E, Rosemary^C, Thyme^E, Yarrow^C

Valley fever

Oils: Basic Vitality Supplements, Cinnamon Bark, Melaleuca **Blends:** Massage Blend, Protective Blend

Note: We have not found an essential oils protocol documented to help with valley fever. Suggestions below are based on symptom relief, core strength and fungal infection in lungs.

Immune system/energy level: Basic Vitality Supplements, the

Massage Blend Technique daily if possible, Energy & Stamina Complex supplement.

Fungal infection: 2-4 drops Protective Blend supplemented with 1-2 drops each Cinnamon Bark and Melaleuca. Diffuse as many hours as possible per day. Prepare an inhaler, use often, breathe deep. Inhale the Respiratory Blend before inhaler. Also cup & inhale technique or in capsules daily.

Symptoms: Headaches, muscle and joint pain use protocols mentioned under those subjects.

Other oils: Clove, Oregano, Rosemary, Thyme **Blends/Products:** Energy & Stamina Complex

Valvular heart disease   *see* Heart conditions

Varicose veins (and Spider veins)
[Varicose ulcers or Venous ulcers]

Oils: Cypress^{EC}, Helichrysum^C, Lavender^C, Lemon^{EC}

Protocol 1: 40-60 drops Helichrysum in 6-8 oz lotion base (Hand & Body Lotion or VCO) topically 2x daily for 6 weeks. Can be combined with protocol below. *see also* Lotion.

Protocol 2: 30 drops Cypress, 20 drops Lavender, 10 drops Lemon (or any citrus oil) in 2 oz lotion base (Hand & Body Lotion or VCO) 2x daily for 1 month, then 1x daily for 3-4 months.

Other oils: Frankincense^C, Geranium^C, Lemongrass^C, Peppermint^C, Yarrow^C **Blends:** Invigorating Blend^C

VCO (Virgin Coconut Oil)   *see EVCO*

Vegan products

Pure essential oils are by nature vegan. Veggie capsules are availble. Some supplements associated with essential oils are vegan-friendly as well.
see Basic Vitality Supplements
see Digestive Blend products
see Metabolic Blend Trim Kit

Vegetable cleaning *see* Household care

Veins, clots *see* Blood clots

Vertigo *(balance)*

Oils: Frankincense, Ginger[C], Helichrysum[C] **Blends:** Basic Vitality Supplements

Prevention: Basic Vitality Supplements, 2-3 drops Ginger topically around ear and bottoms of feet and/or in a capsule internally.

Relief from attack: 1-2 drops of Helichrysum topically on bone behind ear or 2 drops Frankincense under tongue, followed with an additional drop after 30 minutes.

Other oils: Basil[EC], Lavender[EC], Peppermint[C], Ylang Ylang[C]

Vetiver *(Vetiveria zizanoides)*

essential**⬤**oil

Properties: Antibiotic, antimicrobial, antioxidant, antiseptic

Addresses: acne, ADD/ADHD, anger, anxiety, aphrodisiac, arthritis, circulation, mature skin, rheumatism, sedative, stress

(see Safety Chart, page 23)

Viral gastroenteritis *see* Stomach flu

Viral infections *see* Antiviral

AIDS	*see* AIDS
Bronchitis	*see* Bronchitis
Chicken Pox (Shingles)	*see* Chicken Pox
Common cold	*see* Common cold
Conjunctivitis (pink eye)	*see* Conjunctivitis
Influenza	*see* Influenza
Meningitis	*see* Meningitis
Mononucleosis	*see* Mononucleosis
Mumps	*see* Mumps
Rabies (Animal bites)	*see* Rabies

Tonsillitis	*see* Tonsillitis
Warts	*see* Warts

Vision, improve   *see* Eyesight failing

Vitiligo

Oils: Bergamot[C], Black Pepper, Frankincense[C] **Blends/Products:** Basic Vitality Supplements, Cellular Complex Blend, GI Cleansing Formula/ Probiotic Defense Formula

Some success with topical application of Bergamot to affected areas 1-2x daily. Caution: Avoid sunlight, Bergamot is photosensitive.

It may be autoimmune related, *see* Autoimmune.

Basic Vitality Supplements, 1 capsule Cellular Complex Blend 2x daily, 2-3 drops Frankincense 2-4x daily under tongue, GI Cleansing Formula/ Probiotic Defense Formula and Detoxification Blend (*see* Detoxification) and the Massage Blend Technique periodically.

New research suggests Black Pepper but no reported protocols using the essential oil yet.

Other oils: Myrrh[C], Sandalwood[C], Vetiver[C] **Blends:** Cleansing Blend[C], Detoxification Blend, Massage Blend

Vomiting

Oils: Cardamom[EC], Coriander[C], Ginger[EC] **Blends:** Digestive Blend[C]

1-5 drops Digestive Blend or other oils mentioned. Inhale from bottle or inhaler, sip with water or juice, take in capsule or apply topically on abdomen.

Children: Topically with carrier oil on abdomen.

Small infants: Topically to bottoms of feet.

Repeat as soon as 10-15 minutes if necessary for relief.

Other oils: Fennel[E], Peppermint[EC], Roman Chamomile[EC], Rose[EC]

Legend: Preferred, Suggested, Consider

Warts
see also Genital warts

[Common, Flat Molluscum, Plantar, Periungual warts]

Oils: Frankincense^C, Melaleuca^C, Oregano^C **Blends:** Protective Blend^C

Common, plantar, flat, and periungal warts: 1 drop each Oregano and Frankincense (a carrier oil is recommended for children). Apply 2-3x daily on wart and surrounding area, 2-4 weeks or until wart is gone, continue after for 1 week.

Molluscum warts: 2-3 drops Protective Blend or Oregano to bottoms of feet 2-3x daily.

Other oils: Arborvitae^C, Cinnamon Bark^C, Clove^C, Cypress^C, Lemon^EC, Thyme^C **Blends:** Cleansing Blend

Wasp stings
see Bee stings

Water purification

Oils: Lemon^EC

Short term: For antibacterial protection add 1-2 drops Lemon per glass of water or 3-5 drops per gallon.

Emergency preparedness (long-term storage): Use good containers, scrub with Lemon essential oil, fill with filtered, boiled or water from a municipal source (purified). Add 3-5 drops Lemon essential oil to storage water (citrus oils have a finite lifetime, consider rotating yearly) and also add to water at time of use as shown above.

Other oils: Peppermint^C **Blends:** Cleansing Blend^C

Water retention
see Edema

Weakness
see Fatigue, physical

Weight loss

[appetite suppressant, obesity]

Cellulite loss   *see* Skin conditions with weight loss
Skin conditions   *see* Skin conditions with weight loss

OILS:

Basic: Basic Vitality Supplements, Cinnamon Bark, Ginger[C], Grapefruit[C], Lemon[C], Metabolic Blend Trim Shake, Peppermint

Appetite suppressant: Dill[C], Grapefruit[C], Metabolic Blend[C], Patchouli[C]

Attitude: Grounding Blend, Joyful Blend[C], Lavender, Peppermint, Ylang Ylang

Diuretic: Cypress[EC], Fennel[EC], Lavender[EC], Lemon[C], Oregano[C], Rosemary[EC]

Fat burn: Basil, Cypress, Grapefruit[C], Lavender

Metabolism: Eucalyptus, Grapefruit, Peppermint, Rosemary

PROTOCOLS:

Basic nutrition: Use Basic Vitality Supplements consistently.

Suppress appetite: 2-8 drops Metabolic Blend in 16 oz water, sip during day or 5-8 drops in capsule daily.

125 calorie meal: Metabolic Blend shake to replace 1 meal per day.

Reduce cellulites: 2-4 drops Grapefruit, wait 30 sec, 2-4 drops Metabolic Blend topically to cellulite areas.

Cleansing: Under Detoxification *see* Nutritional cleanses and Isolated cleanses/Gastrointestinal tract.

Note: When choosing any of the oils above please review all of the safety precautions on pages 23-28.

Weight management   *see* Metabolic Blend and Metabolic Trim Kit

West Nile   *see* Flu

Western Red Cedar   *see* **Arborvitae**

Whiplash   *see* Back conditions

White Fir *(Albies alba)*

essential oil

Properties: Antibiotic, antioxidant, antiseptic, astringent, disinfectant, diuretic

Addresses: Arthritic pain, cold and flu, congestion, immune strengthener, infections, joint pain, muscle pain

(see Safety Chart, page 23)

Whooping cough

Oils: Cypress[EC], Eucalyptus, Frankincense, Lemongrass, Oregano[EC], Thyme[EC] **Blends:** Protective Blend, Respiratory Blend

Adults: 5 drops Protective Blend, 2 drops each Frankincense and Oregano in capsule, 2x daily.

Children/infants: Layer on the chest with carrier oil 1-2 drops each Thyme, then Cypress, then Eucalyptus, follow with warm compress. Repeat every 1-3 hours. Also alternate 1-2 drops Protective Blend and Oregano on bottoms of feet.

Everyone: Diffuse Respiratory Blend and Lemongrass often. Digestive Blend for nausea and vomiting.

Other oils: Basil[EC], Clary Sage[EC], Grapefruit[C], Lavender[EC], Lime, Ravensara

Wild Orange *(Citrus sinensis)*

essential oil

Properties: Antibacterial, antidepressant, antifungal, anti-inflammatory, antioxidant, antiseptic, carminative, choleretic, digestive, hypotensive, sedative, stimulant

Addresses: Acid reflux, cold and flu, depression, heartburn, indigestion, muscle pain, stomachache, stress

(see Safety Chart, page 23)

Wintergreen *(Gaultheria fragrantissima)*

essential oil [sourced from Nepal]

Properties: similar to Gaultheria procubens (see next item) but said to be "warmer", much like Birch oil

Addresses: Arthritic pain, joint pain, soothing, stimulating, uplifting

(see Safety Chart, page 23)

Wintergreen *(Gaultheria procumbens)*

essential oil [sourced from China, often used in blends such as a Soothing Blend]

Properties: Analgesic, anti-inflammatory, antiseptic, astringent

Addresses: Arthritic pain, dermatitis, joint pain, skin disorders

(see Safety Chart, page 23)

Women's Monthly Blend   *see* Monthly Blend for Women

Women's Phytoestrogen Complex   *see* Phytoestrogen complex

Worms   *see* Parasite infections

Wounds   *see* Cuts and wounds

Wrinkles *(and facial fine lines)*

Oils: Frankincense^C, Geranium^C, Helichrysum^C, Lavender^C **Blends/Products:** Anti-Aging Blend^C, Anti-Aging Moisturizer, Tightening Serum (*see* Skin care)

Moisturize with Anti-Aging Moisturizer or equivalent oils with EVCO (Lavender, Geranium, and Frankincense) and tighten with Tightening Serum or equivalent oils (Frankincense, Sandalwood and Myrrh).

Other oils: Copaiba^C, Elemi^C, Jasmine^C, Myrrh^C, Neroli^C, Sandalwood^C

Yarrow (Achilea nobilis)

essential oil

Properties: Anti-inflammatory. antiseptic, antispasmodic, astringent, digestive stimulant

Addresses: Acne, agitation, alopecia, amenorrhoea, arthritis, cellulitis, colds, congestion, cuts, eczema, fever, flatulence, gall bladder inflammation, gastriris, gout, headache, hemorrhoids, high blood pressure, hormonal balance, insect bites, loss of appetitie, kidney infection, nausea, oligomenorrhea, PMS, prostatitis, scar reduction, sprains, stomachaches, UTI, vaginitis, varicose veins

(see Safety Chart, page 23)

Yarrow-Pomegranate Blend

essential oils
Blend

Ingredients: Pomegranate seed oil, Yarrow

Addresses: Aging skin, an antioxidant, anxiety (calming), healthy metabolism, immune system support, release fatty acids, skin blemishes, skin care

(see Safety Chart, page 23)

Yeast infection
see Candida

Yellow jacket bite/sting
see Bee stings

Ylang Ylang (Cananga ordorata)

essential oil

Properties: Antidepressant, antiseptic, antispasmodic, sedative

Addresses: Depression, dermatitis, hair care, hypertension, indigestion, insomnia, skin disorders, stomachache, stress

Yoga Blends

essential oils
Blend

Centering, Enlightening and Steadying essential oil blends coupled with yoga moves and poses can bring improved harmony and purpose to life.

Notes:

Legend: Preferred, Suggested, Consider

Helpful Charts

On the following pages are included charts that will help in the use of essential oils. You will find:

- Reflexology Charts - Foot, Hand and Ear diagrams show the specific points that are associated with the major organs and areas of the body. Many find these as useful locations to apply oils to strengthen or help the associated body part.

  - ◆ Bottoms of feet chart
  - ◆ Tops of feet chart
  - ◆ Hand chart
  - ◆ Ear chart

- Massage-like techniques to apply essential oils.

  - ◆ Massage Blend Technique "Reminder Chart" gives a visual summary of the Massage Blend Technique. The chart may be used during application as a handy reminder of what oils and what strokes are to be used during each of the phases of this procedure.

  - ◆ Massage Blend Hand Technique is a simplfied way to get the benefits of the full Massage Blend Technique in the previous chart.

  - ◆ Baby Foot Massage suggestions.

- How many drops? - A quick reference help to determine how many drops are in a bottle, can be put in a capsule, etc.

- A list of the generic blend names used in this book and space to list your favorite name for that same blend.

Reflexology Foot Chart I

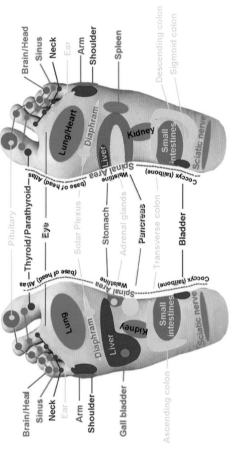

Bottom Right Foot

Bottom Left Foot

© 2015 Essentials of the Earth, LLC

These reflexology maps are based on the concept that the ear, foot, or hand are connected to all the other parts of the body through the nervous system or "energy" system and thus become a reflection or snapshot of the entire body. These charts were developed by comparing a number of Chinese and other mappings and looking for the commonality among them. They can generally be regarded as a merging of Chinese mappings with additions from the more recent French studies. It has been the experience of those using essential oils that applying oils to the pressure points identified by other disciplines (reflexology, acupressure, acupuncture and massage) can provide another "gateway" to various parts of the body.

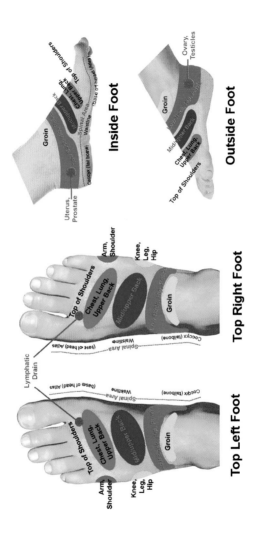

Reflexology Foot Chart II

Inside Foot

Top of Shoulders
Upper Back
Chest, Lung,
Spinal Area
Waistline
Base of head/Atlas
Coccyx (tail bone)
Groin
Uterus, Prostate

Outside Foot

Ovary, Testicles
Groin
Midplantar Band
Chest, Lung, Upper Back
Top of Shoulders

Top Right Foot

Arm, Shoulder
Knee, Leg, Hip
Top of Shoulders
Chest, Lung, Upper Back
Midplantar Band
Groin
Atlas (base of head)
Waistline
Spinal Area
Coccyx (tailbone)

Top Left Foot

Lymphatic Drain
Atlas (base of head)
Waistline
Spinal Area
Coccyx (tailbone)
Top of Shoulders
Chest, Lung, Upper Back
Midplantar Band
Groin
Arm, Shoulder
Knee, Leg, Hip

Safety charts ... page 23   Special cautions ... page 3

Reflexology Hand Chart

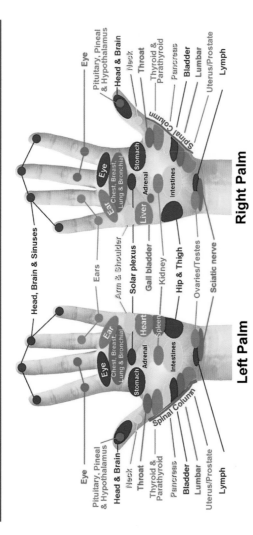

Left Palm

Right Palm

Head, Brain & Sinuses

Eye
Pituitary, Pineal & Hypothalamus
Head & Brain
Neck
Throat
Thyroid & Parathyroid
Pancreas
Bladder
Lumbar
Uterus/Prostate
Lymph

Eye
Pituitary, Pineal & Hypothalamus
Head & Brain
Neck
Throat
Thyroid & Parathyroid
Pancreas
Bladder
Lumbar
Uterus/Prostate
Lymph

Ears
Arm & Shoulder
Solar plexus
Gall bladder
Kidney
Hip & Thigh
Ovaries/Testes
Sciatic nerve

Eye
Ear
Chest, Breast, Lung & Bronchial
Stomach
Adrenal
Heart
Spleen
Intestines
Liver
Spinal Column

These reflexology maps are based on the concept that the ear, foot, or hand are connected to all the other parts of the body through the nervous system or "energy" system and thus become a reflection or snapshot of the entire body. These charts were developed by comparing a number of Chinese and other mappings and looking for the commonality among them. They can generally be regarded as a merging of Chinese mappings with additions from the more recent French studies. It has been the experience of those using essential oils that applying oils to the pressure points identified by other disciplines (reflexology, acupressure, acupuncture and massage) can provide another "gateway" to various parts of the body.

Reflexology Ear Chart

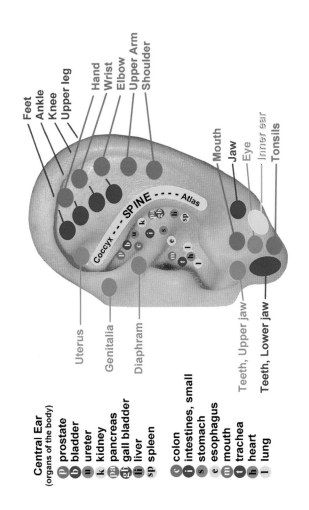

© 2015 Essentials of the Earth, LLC

Feet
Ankle
Knee
Upper leg

Hand
Wrist
Elbow
Upper Arm
Shoulder

Mouth
Jaw
Eye
Inner ear
Tonsils

SPINE · · · · Atlas
Coccyx

Uterus
Genitalia
Diaphram

Teeth, Upper jaw
Teeth, Lower jaw

Central Ear
(organs of the body)
- p prostate
- b bladder
- u ureter
- k kidney
- pa pancreas
- gb gall bladder
- li liver
- sp spleen

- c colon
- i intestines, small
- s stomach
- e esophagus
- m mouth
- t trachea
- h heart
- l lung

Massage Blend Technique
A CLINICAL APPROACH TO ESSENTIAL OIL APPLICATION

The Massage Blend Blend Technique was developed by leading experts on the use of essential oils for improving wellness. The technique was created to manage four systemic constants that are common factors in overall wellness. These factors are: stress, toxic insult, inflammatory response and autonomic imbalance.

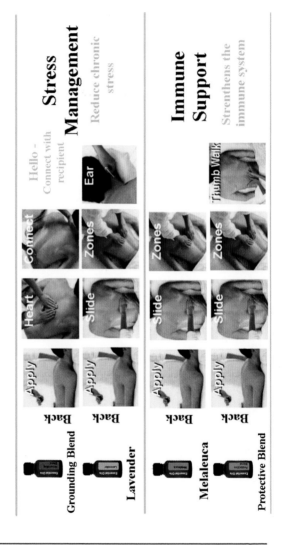

Stress Management — Reduce chronic stress

Immune Support — Strenthens the immune system

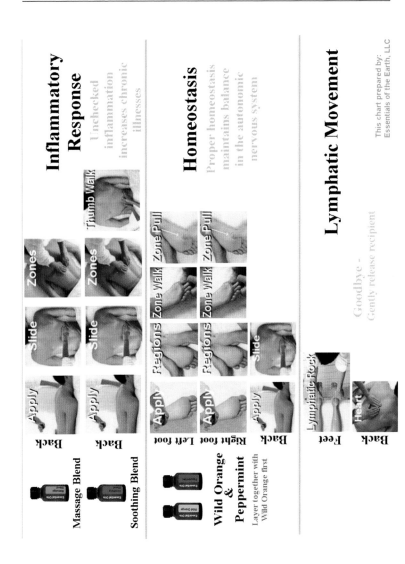

Inflammatory Response

Unchecked inflammation increases chronic illnesses

Back — Apply, Slide, Zones
Back — Apply, Slide, Zones, Thumb Walk

Massage Blend

Soothing Blend

Homeostasis

Proper homeostasis maintains balance in the autonomic nervous system

Right foot — Apply, Regions, Zone Walk, Zone Pull
Left foot — Apply, Regions, Zone Walk, Zone Pull
Back — Apply, Slide

Wild Orange & Peppermint

Layer together with Wild Orange first

Lymphatic Movement

Goodbye - Gently release recipient

Feet — Lymphatic Rock
Back — Heart

This chart prepared by: Essentials of the Earth, LLC

Massage Blend Hand Technique

The Massage Blend Hand Technique gives you a way to give many of the benefits of the full body Massage Blend Technique in a more convenient way. No massage table or privacy is required. Makes it possible to share with physically limited folks and with anyone in a home meeting, a show or other public locations. Follow the six steps below:

The Preparation Steps

Step 1
Use both hands to grip one of the recipient's hands on either side with the dorsum (back) of their hand facing upward and with your thumbs on top.

Step 2
Use your thumbs to stretch the tissue of the hand moving from the inside to the outward edge, and from their wrist to the base of the fingers.

Step 3
Turn the recipient's hand over and apply a light, even coating of your selected oil, oils or blend to the entire palm side of the hand.

The After-Oils Steps

Step 4
Grip the recipient's hand with one hand on either side, with your thumbs on top. Use your thumbs to methodically work through the hand's 3 regions, beginning in region 1, with medium pressure. Make sure to massage the entire surface area of each of the hand's regions.

Step 5
Next, use your thumbs to work through each of the hand's 5 zones. Beginning in zone 1, place your thumbs at the top of the recipient's hand close to the wrist and alternately work thumbs down the entire length of zone 1 to the tip of the finger. Repeat the procedure for all 5 zones.

Step 6
Finally do an inter-phalangeal pull by putting the recipient's palm facing up, grip their wrist in one hand. Use your other hand to stretch the inter-Phalangeal tissue, the tissue located between each finger, away from their hand by gripping and sliding the tissue between your thumb and forefinger. Repeat the pull three times in-between each finger before moving on to the next.

Repeat the complete procedure for the other hand.

Regions

Zones

Inter-phalangeal Pull

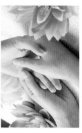

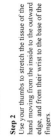

Baby Foot Massage

Help your baby with light massage using soothing strokes and light pressure. Coupling this with appropriate diluted essential oils can be so helpful to a baby's care. It is also comforting to the parent as well. Consider below the different zones of the foot and how they reflect areas that may need occasional attention on your baby.

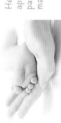

Hold the baby's foot in your hands and apply gentle pressure and strokes in the different areas described below for relaxing comfort and benefits to both baby and parent.

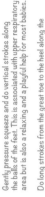

Gently squeezing individually the tips of the toes and massaging/squeezing the great toe focuses on the head, teeth and sinuses. Consider for congestion or teething.

Gently pressure squeeze and do vertical strokes along the balls of the feet. This is associated with upper respiratory area but is also a relaxing and a playful help for most babies.

Do long strokes from the great toe to the heel along the arch area. This is associated with the spine and is also a very relaxing and calming motion for most babies.

Apply gentle pressure and circular motions on the arch and mid-foot. This is the primary area for digestive discomforts.

Address the heel areas with gentle thumb pressure from spot to spot. Use this to relax and also for digestive discomforts.

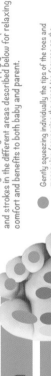

Head/Teeth

Sinus area

Upper abdomen

Lower abdomen

Pelvic area

Safety charts ... page 23   Special cautions ... page 3

Quick Reference for "How Many Drops Are ...?"

How many drops are in common containers?

Container	Drops (average)
1 ml	20
5 ml bottle is same as 1 teaspoon	85 (minimum) 100 (average)
15 ml bottle is same as 1 Tablespoon	250 (minimum) 300 (average)
1 oz	600

How many drops in a bottle of ... ?

Essential Oil	Drops in 5 ml (ave)
Lemon	85
Melaleuca	87
Oregano	120
Frankincense	124
Sandalwood	135
Peppermint	140

How many drops in a capsule?

Capsule size	# of mg	# of drops
00 capsule	735	15-20
0 capsule	500	10-13

How many drops do I add to a teaspoon of VCO to have a ... % mixture?

Carrier/ Mixture	1%	2%	5%	10%
1 teaspoon	1 drop	2 drops	5 drops	10 drops
1 Tablespoon	3 drops	6 drops	15 drops	30 drops
1 fluid oz	6 drops	12 drops	30 drops	60 drops

Essential Oils Blends

Generic Name	My Product Name
Anti-Aging Blend	
Blend for Women	
Cellular Complex	
Centering Blend (Yoga help)	
Cleansing Blend	
Comforting Blend (Emotional help)	
Courage Blend for Children	
Detoxification Blend	
Digestive Blend	
Encouraging Blend (Emotional help)	
Enlightening Blend (Yoga help)	
Fortifying Blend	
Focus Blend	
Focus Blend for Children	
Grounding Blend	
Grounding Blend for Children	
Inspiring Blend (Emotional help)	
Invigorating Blend	
Joyful Blend	
Massage Blend	
Metabolic Blend	
Monthly Blend for Women (formerly Women's Monthly Blend)	
Outdoor Blend (formerly Repellent)	
Protective Blend	
Protective Blend for Children	
Reassuring Blend (Emotional help)	
Renewing Blend (Emotional help)	
Respiratory Blend	
Restful Blend (formerly Calming)	
Restful Blend for Children	

Safety charts ... page 23   Special cautions ... page 3

Seasonal Blend	
Soothing Blend	
Soothing Blend for Children	
Steadying Blend (Yoga help)	
Tension Blend	
Topical Blend	
Uplifting Blend (Emotional help)	
Yarrow-Pomegranate Blend	

Notes: